T0044582

WORK OUT

ALSO BY JASON KARP

Running Periodization
Track & Field Omnibook (Editor)
The Inner Runner
Running a Marathon For Dummies
Lose It Forever
Sexercise
Running for Women
Run Your Fat Off
14-Minute Metabolic Workouts
101 Winning Racing Strategies for Runners
101 Developmental Concepts & Workouts for Cross Country Runners
How to Survive Your PhD

WORK OUT

The Revolutionary Method of Creating a Sound Body to Create a Sound Mind

JASON R. KARP, PHD, MBA

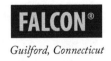

Guilford, Connecticut

An imprint of The Rowman & Littlefield Publishing Group, Inc.
4501 Forbes Blvd., Ste. 200
Lanham, MD 20706
www.rowman.com

Falcon and FalconGuides are registered trademarks and Make Adventure Your Story is a trademark of The Rowman & Littlefield Publishing Group, Inc.

Distributed by NATIONAL BOOK NETWORK

Copyright © 2022 Jason R. Karp, PhD, MBA

All rights reserved. No part of this book may be reproduced in any form or by any electronic or mechanical means, including information storage and retrieval systems, without written permission from the publisher, except by a reviewer who may quote passages in a review.

British Library Cataloguing in Publication Information available

Library of Congress Cataloging-in-Publication Data available
Names: Karp, Jason, author.
Title: Work out : the revolutionary method of creating a sound body to create a sound mind / Jason R. Karp.
Description: Guilford, Connecticut : FalconGuides, 2022. | Includes bibliographical references and index. | Summary: "A fitness guide that takes an outside-in approach to show how strengthening the body first leads to a stronger mind and inner self, explaining how exercise creates the sound mind and changes us on the inside and then by describing the workouts to create the sound body"— Provided by publisher.
Identifiers: LCCN 2021043015 (print) | LCCN 2021043016 (ebook) | ISBN 9781493060979 (paperback) | ISBN 9781493060986 (epub)
Subjects: LCSH: Exercise—Psychological aspects. | Physical fitness—Psychological aspects. | Mind and body.
Classification: LCC GV481.2 .K37 2022 (print) | LCC GV481.2 (ebook) | DDC 613.7/1—dc23
LC record available at https://lccn.loc.gov/2021043015
LC ebook record available at https://lccn.loc.gov/2021043016

♾ The paper used in this publication meets the minimum requirements of American National Standard for Information Sciences—Permanence of Paper for Printed Library Materials, ANSI/NISO Z39.48-1992.

The author and The Rowman & Littlefield Publishing Group, Inc., assume no liability for accidents happening to, or injuries sustained by, readers who engage in the activities described in this book.

*To my dad, Monroe, whose heart attack that took his life
taught me the importance of training my heart.*

*And to my mom, Muriel, whose love of sports and career
as a physical education teacher influenced me to become
an athlete and a student of athletics.*

They are with me with every step I run.

Contents

Acknowledgments

WHILE WRITING A BOOK IS SOLITARY WORK, MANY PEOPLE ARE involved in the process and deserve mention. At the top of that list is my literary agent, Grace Freedson. If not for her, publishers may never read my book proposals. It has been fourteen years since receiving her typewritten letter in my self-addressed stamped envelope, in which she offered to represent me and my work. It was the only piece of mail I received that day, on my final day of receiving mail before moving to another part of the country. I thank her for taking a chance.

When I write a book, I think about the process my twin brother and playwright, Jack Karp, takes when he writes a play, planning out the play's structure and outline of each scene on paper, then adroitly piecing the scenes together to create both a captivating story and a piece of art. Jack is the best writer I know. He inspires me every day to view writing as art and explained to me, in the words of Hemingway, "the first draft of anything is shit" and should be thrown out. The first draft of this book was indeed thrown out, replaced with a new vision and table of contents that read nothing like the one in my original book proposal.

Thank you to the publishing and editorial team at Globe Pequot, including editor David Legere, production editor Meredith Dias, and copy editor Lauren Szalkiewicz, for shaping this book into something that I hope will help people see themselves in a new light, as the physical animals we are. I am grateful to Globe

Pequot for the opportunity to publicly share my thoughts, ideas, and words.

The idea for this book started as an idea for a TED talk, which I was asked to give at TEDxRexburg in Rexburg, Idaho. I am grateful to the team at TEDxRexburg, who believed my idea worth spreading was worthy of the TED stage.

Finally, if not for the scientists whose research traverses several disciplines, including evolutionary biology, anatomy, neurobiology, psychology, and exercise physiology, this book would have been merely a rant of my personal musings as a runner. It is the scientists' creative research that has elucidated the embodied life and how our inside Mind is affected by our outside Body. I hope this book does their research justice.

Prologue

Inscribed on the off-white parchment of my PhD diploma is the vague term "human performance." When people ask me about the degree, I tell them it is in exercise physiology, since that was the specific subject I studied. Saying that I did a PhD in human performance would likely cause some confused looks, which would require that I clarify. And to do that, I would first need to come up with a clarification of human performance for myself.

While working on the degree, I was asked to write a research paper on evolution and the limits of human athletic performance. It was a difficult paper to write. I wrote about such things as natural selection, genetic drift and gene flow, divergence of character, aerobic metabolic capacity, Body mass, the quantities of useful muscular force and mechanical power that can be generated and sustained, and an esoteric anatomical theory called *symmorphosis*.

Symmorphosis proposes that an organism's structural design is regulated by its functional demand.[1,2] Perhaps the most prominent promoter of symmorphosis is preeminent anatomist Ewald Weibel, MD, who wrote, "the quantity of structure incorporated into an animal's functional system is matched to what is needed: enough but not too much."[3] Thus, it is *demand* that drives the change in an organism's *structure*. Any extra baggage is not supported and becomes extinct. The human Body can change, and the limits of human performance can only be exceeded, if the demand on the Body's performance increases.

While symmorphosis is quite a long process, occurring on a species level over millions of years of evolution, structural changes also occur on an individual level in the short term (weeks to months in your lifetime) in response to specific stressors, physical exercise being the most prolific and potent one. In response to physical exercise, muscle fibers increase their metabolic machinery, bones increase their density, cardiac muscle enlarges, new blood vessels sprout around muscle fibers, and new neurons are formed in the Brain. These changes are quite sensitive to imposed stresses. Indeed, your Body (and the structure of all organisms) evolves to cope with all but the most extreme stresses to which it is subjected.

If the quantity of structure incorporated into an individual's system is matched to what is needed, increasing the need through physical training increases the amount of change that takes place. However, changes are not limited to anatomical structures and functions, as symmorphosis proposes; other functions change as well, including cognition, mindset, and confidence. These functions go way beyond symmorphosis.

Physical training is quite a remarkable process. And what it proves is that we are not static creatures. Not physically and not psychologically. Human performance is ever-changing, and we have control over the degree to which we change.

No matter how I define human performance to others and to myself, every definition I come up with concerns the Body. Because the human existence and the human experience are physical.

My passion for human performance began during the Presidential Physical Fitness Tests in fifth grade. Two of the tests were a 50-yard sprint in the school's parking lot and a 600-yard run on the grass field. I ran the former in 7.3 seconds and the latter in

2 minutes and 1 second. It was then that I discovered that I had some talent, although I wasn't the quickest in my class. But I was close. It was also then that I discovered the freedom that running confers, the freedom of all-out physical effort. Little did I know how much it would direct and shape my life.

A year later, during my first formal race of 400 meters on my middle school track team, I became hooked. Running as fast as my legs could, I was free.

Free from the noise of the outside world.

Free from the insecurities of my inside self.

And there was no turning back. Thirty-eight years later, I'm still running six days per week, still running to free myself from the noise and from the insecurities.

It didn't take long after becoming a runner to realize the power of the physical being. When I run fast, when I *feel* fast, it creates a powerful confidence that penetrates everything else I do. I feel on top of the world. Being physically fit influences the way I feel about myself, my outlook on what I can achieve, and who I can be. And the converse is also true—when I'm not fit, when I don't *feel* fast, my confidence wavers. My thoughts are not the same. My ideas are not as malleable, not as expansive, not as open to change.

Being a lifelong runner and coach, I often think about training methods. I have even written several books on the subject. I think and research a lot about training the Body, more than anyone I know. Running is all physical, so there's little else to think about. Other sports have attributes other than the pure physical act. In football, for example, coaches and players spend a lot of time analyzing their opponent's plays by watching films of games, dissecting each scenario and the teams' corresponding inclinations. From that analysis, they develop defensive and offensive strategies to win the upcoming game. Running, by contrast, is a lot simpler. While there are strategies involved, especially at the elite level and during longer races, the person who wins is usually the one who is the fastest, at least on that day. And speed and endurance are physical attributes.

And so I spend a lot of time thinking about how runners can get faster. I spend a lot of time thinking about the physical.

But running is not just about getting faster. Not really.

When we recognize that ideas are embodied, and that the Body can change with training, we don't allow our ideas to become dogmas. Like the scientist who changes his or her ideas through the diligent and consistent testing of hypotheses, ideas can be molded, ideas can be influenced, ideas can be changed by training the Body. We change the Body and we change our thoughts and our ideas and our Minds.

As far back as the ancient Greeks and Romans, humans understood the relationship between the physical and the psychological, between the Body and the Mind. Most people have heard of the famous phrase "a sound Mind in a sound Body," which was coined by the Roman poet Juvenal when he wrote around the end of the first century AD, *"Orandum est ut sit mens sana in corpore sano"*—"We should pray for a healthy Mind in a healthy Body."

Over 2,000 years later, we struggle with the dualism of Mind and Body.

We have lost our way.

We have forgotten that we are animals.

We like to think of ourselves as different from other animals, that we possess special qualities that distinguish us from our pets. But when we think about what is special about us, we must remember that the characteristics that make humans special are built upon a physical, biological foundation that is shared with many other animals.

Somewhere between chasing other animals for food and clicking a mouse to purchase a toaster oven on Amazon.com, we stopped living a physical life. Instead, we are encouraged to work on our inner selves, to practice mindfulness, to meditate, and to get our minds right, whatever "right" means. Social media gives us

"Monday motivation" and shouts daily positivity. Law of attraction followers say that our thoughts directly change our lives, that we can manifest what we want from the universe. Parents, teachers, Olympic athletes, and practically everyone else tell us that we can achieve anything that we set our minds to. Many books are written about mindset and how our minds can control everything, from our love lives to cancerous tumor growth. Prominent people tell us to start from our *why* and look inward to live our best life.

But that's all wrong. Or, at least, incomplete.

We are physical animals first.

And our physical, animal bodies can change and adapt to different stimuli, causing profound changes to our Brains and affecting our Minds.

All it takes is an increase in the physical demand.

━━━

While the writing of *Work Out* took several months, the central idea behind the words on these pages took many years to develop and manifest, only after spending many years running six days per week, finally arriving at the point that I could satisfactorily articulate and share them. What makes *Work Out* a revolutionary approach is that it runs counter to what society promulgates. It breaks apart the Mind-Body *dualism* that places the Mind ahead of the Body, and treats it as the Body-Mind *dependence* that places the Body ahead of the Mind. I think that is an idea worth spreading.

This book is based on my March 2022 TED talk, *How Running Like an Animal Makes Us Human*, which was postponed several times due to the COVID-19 pandemic, its threat to our physical health and to our lives serving as yet another reminder of the bodily nature of the human existence.

PART I

THE *WORK OUT* APPROACH

"Is this a slippery slope?" I asked the doctor in the hallway of the hospital.

We were standing about 10 feet away from my mother's corner room at the end of the long hallway, the vinyl tile floor feeling hard on my legs after my morning run. Inside the room, my mother lay in the white starch-sheeted bed, in pain from bone cancer, which had metastasized from the breast cancer that had been diagnosed twelve years earlier. She had just returned to the room from an ultrasound that revealed bilateral deep vein thrombosis—blood clots in both of her legs.

"Yes," the doctor replied, solemnly.

I looked out the hallway window that overlooked the parking lot, the red maple and pitch pine trees off in the distance, to collect my thoughts and emotions.

For the next two weeks, I sat with my twin brother by our mother's bedside, holding her hands until all was literally said and done. It was the most emotional experience I've ever had. What was particularly difficult was to watch my mom's physical decline and how it affected her Mind and, ultimately, her will to live. When I made the trip from San Diego to New Jersey two weeks earlier, I never thought I would be planning a funeral. I didn't pack a suit.

In her youth and for many of her adult years, my mom lived a physical life. She was a tough physical education teacher from the Bronx. She competed in the roller derby. She skydived. She played semi-professional softball with her iconic four-fingered glove (she had five fingers like everyone else, but baseball gloves in those days had only four). She raised twin sons as a single mother after our father passed away when we were 8 years old. And she physically cared for her own elderly mother, who was her best friend.

Every day over the final two weeks of my mother's life, I ran every morning before going to the hospital. Sometimes, I ran in the dark at night after leaving. I ran to find myself and to gain the strength that I needed for my mother. And for myself. Running gives us an enormous amount of strength.

Why? Why does running give us strength?

I have spent nearly four decades working on the answer. I even had to write this whole book to explain it to myself.

Apart from its numerous well-documented health and aesthetic benefits, physical conditioning, whether running, weight training, or something else that enables us to push our physical boundaries, changes us on the inside. It strengthens our belief in ourselves and what we can do. It fills the hole created by insecurity.

This transformation starts with physical conditioning.

This transformation isn't some pseudo-holistic platitude, with false promises that making bigger biceps makes you confident and successful.

It's science.

By working on the outside, you can actually alter your physiology, change your Brain chemistry, and change your outlook on life . . . and on yourself.

Many scientific studies have shown that exercise causes profound changes on the inside that positively affect your creativity, your cognition, and your confidence, from the opioids and cannabinoids released in the Brain that cause a perceived euphoria—the "runner's high"—to the increase in serotonin that makes exercise even more effective than prescription drugs for ameliorating depression, to the formation of new neurons in the Brain that changes the way you think. Cardiovascular exercise, such as running and cycling, has also been shown to mitigate symptoms of attention-deficit/hyperactivity disorder (ADHD) in children and adults. The changes that exercise causes happen even down to the tiniest of your Body's cells, where the business of life occurs, and the nucleic acids and bases that create the helical strands of your DNA.

These changes all start by working *out*.

Workout is a relatively new word in the English language, coming into use around 1894. First used in relation to boxing training, it has come to mean more generally an exercise to test or improve one's fitness for athletic competition or human performance. Its verb form, *work out*, is much older, dating back to 1534, and means to bring about by labor and exertion. Thus, to work out is to improve performance by labor and exertion.

When you work out, you create a sound external, which creates a sound internal.

You create a sound Body, which creates a sound Mind.

When you create a sound Body, which creates a sound Mind, you are enabled and empowered to live the life you want, the life you care about, the life you desire.

Your life doesn't start from the inside. It starts from the outside. Because you are an animal.

———

In the couple years prior to running in the 2008 US Olympic Marathon Trials in New York, Jon was training in Kansas City, Missouri, where he was attending law school. He ran 90 to 100 miles per week on a regular basis, one week running more than 120 miles, and ran twice per day nearly every day while juggling classes on legal reasoning and civil procedure and spending countless hours in the law library. His alarm was set for 5:30 a.m. for his morning runs.

When his alarm buzzed, Jon didn't hit the snooze button like many other people do. Instead, he rolled himself out of bed and fell onto the hardwood floor, a rather atypical ritual to wake himself up and get out the door. "Once I hit the floor, I knew I would get out of bed," he says matter-of-factly. It was dark and 20 degrees outside.

Jon grew up running. He had been a very good runner in high school, running a mile in 4:19 and 2 miles in 9:42, and then ran in college on two NCAA Division I teams, running 8:25 for 3,000 meters and 14:45 for 5K, which are excellent performances for a runner. After college, he continued to train, and would go on to run a 2:21 marathon along the streets of Chicago, which qualified him for the 2008 US Olympic Marathon Trials.

But he wasn't a runner anymore.

When I met with Jon, he had just finished meeting with his last client of the day. An attorney in private practice, he and his law firm partner were very busy with clients and managing a staff of nine employees.

Although he was working a lot, things weren't going as well as Jon had hoped. He wasn't living up to his expectations. He was struggling. He was stressed. He had gained nearly 60 pounds since his days of running 90 miles per week. His work had become work. The work he used to love to do. The work that once brought him joy, fighting legal battles for his clients, navigating the complex legal system, searching for justice.

As I approached him in the lobby of his Indianapolis office building, he stopped walking toward me and half-smiled, as if he were anxious about our meeting. We took the elevator up nineteen floors and sat in his office to talk, the floor-to-ceiling windows overlooking the silver skyscrapers of Monument Circle. His laptop computer sat open in the center of his desk, with several stacks of legal documents and a half-finished can of Coca-Cola a few inches away. It was the most comfortable place for Jon, a place where he felt like home. But lately, it had become a place of stress.

"When I'm not in court, I spend all my time in this office," he said, gesturing to his desk and paperwork. "I should get outside more."

"How are things going?" I asked deliberately, in hopes of getting more than a casual response.

"I feel anxious when I'm not working," he confided, "so I'll work more to relieve my anxiety. When I work, nothing else matters.

"I'm very hard on myself. I feel like I'm always pushing for something, like I did when I was running. But I have no more energy. I'm exhausted every day."

He paused and looked away for a moment, staring outside the window. The late-day sun casted a metallic orange glow on the skyscrapers.

"Sometimes, I'll come back to the office at night, or I'll work on the weekends at home. With all the work I do, I should be moving up the ladder faster. I should be getting bigger clients and making more money. Work is not fun anymore. I feel overwhelmed. I don't know what to do.

"I remember when I first graduated law school ten years ago, I was so excited. I felt so limitless. I want to feel like that free-spirited athlete again who could conquer the world!"

"Jon," I said as encouragingly as I could, "every lawyer works. But it takes more than work to be successful. The work does not give you freedom.

"Every human has three parts: Body, Brain, and Mind. When they work together and are equally balanced, life is great and hums along the way life is supposed to. The Body would be strong, resilient, and enduring, the Brain would be buzzing with electrical activity, and the Mind would be analytical, confident, and emotionally intelligent, navigating challenges and figuring out solutions to problems.

"Unfortunately, few people are blessed with such a balance. Body, Brain, and Mind often work in conflict with one another. They all want to be the boss.

"But there can be only one boss, Jon. Only one boss.

"Think of your law firm. The junior associates of the firm don't just do mindless work. They have a manager—the boss—who strategizes about what's right for the firm, how to make the associates and the firm successful. The manager directs the associates to do the right work that is aligned with the firm's mission to get results. That's what you need to do, Jon, with your own life. And you can do it."

Jon nodded and half-smiled.

"It's easy to spend time thinking, worrying, brewing over the stress and let your thoughts control your life," I said.

"It's easy to tell someone to meditate or to ask what your *why* is.

"You think a lion asks himself, 'What's my *why?*'

"For Christ's sake, no!" I exclaimed. I didn't wait for Jon to answer.

"The lion is the king of the jungle. He acts like the king because he knows no other way. His Body is the boss. He uses his Body every day to intimidate other animals, chase them for lunch, protect his family, and rule over his kingdom.

"Before you use your amazing Mind, Jon, which is capable of thinking and creating on a much higher level than that of a lion, you must first understand where your Mind's thoughts come from, how they are assembled inside your Brain, and how your Brain functions inside your Body."

Jon seemed a bit overwhelmed.

"What does my life have to do with a lion?" he asked. "A lion sleeps, eats, and chases other animals all day. I don't have the time to do any of that," he said, sounding frustrated. "I sit at my desk all day and work harder than anyone else. Then, I go home to my wife and kids. But I feel like my life is falling apart."

"That's just it, Jon," I said. "You sit at your desk all day. Your life has become unbalanced. Your Body was never meant to stop running and sit at your desk all day. Because the Body is the boss. Training the Body changes the Brain, which affects the Mind. Training the Body eliminates the conflict between Body, Brain, and Mind, making all three parts work in harmony.

"You're much more similar to a lion than you think.

"You can find that free-spirited athlete again, Jon, who can conquer the world. All the inspiration and solution you need already reside in you, as they do in every human. You just need to start with your Body.

"Why don't we take a look at how to live the life you want? It's time to learn how creating a sound Body creates a sound Mind."

CHAPTER ONE

Body

THE BODY TALKS TO US AND
GIVES US CLUES TO ITS NEEDS

ON FRIDAY MORNING, 47-YEAR-OLD JILL BRAXMEYER HOLDS A
20-pound dumbbell in each hand like a suitcase, facing a large
mirror at MetroFlex Gym in Oceanside, California, near her
home in Vista. To target the medial head of the deltoid muscle
in her shoulders, she raises both arms laterally until her arms are
parallel to the floor, and then lowers her arms down to her sides,
repeating this movement eight to twelve times. As she slowly and
methodically lifts the dumbbells, the multipennate fibers of her
deltoid muscles create visible striations in the mirror, as if the
muscles had been sculpted by Rodin. At the end of the set, she
rests her shoulders for a minute and then repeats another eight
to twelve reps, continuing this sequence until she completes four
sets of lateral raises, for a total of thirty-two to forty-eight reps.
"I make sure not to lift too heavy so that I don't recruit my traps
(trapezius muscles) because I don't want to build those," she says.

It's the second day this week Jill is training her deltoids. It's
one of the areas of her Body that needs growth, she says. "For
shoulders, you have to target anterior, medial, and posterior heads
of the muscle to create a nice roundness," she says.

Bodybuilders think a lot about muscle size and shape.

Jill typically lifts weights five days per week and does cardio exercise five days per week. She splits her weight training between legs and glutes twice per week and shoulders twice per week. She adds in training of the "pull" muscles of the back and biceps and the "push" muscles of the chest and triceps on the same days that she trains her shoulders.

When she's not lifting weights, Jill is a fitness and nutrition coach and neurofeedback Brain trainer. Neurofeedback is a type of biofeedback that uses displays of Brain activity in real time using non-invasive electroencephalography to teach self-regulation of Brain function. Her clients include individuals who have had head trauma, CEOs, and individuals with sleep issues, attention deficit disorder, depression, anxiety, and those who are grieving a loss.

Jill started lifting weights in high school when she was 15 years old, a year after competing on her school's dance team. It was the early 1990s, when there weren't many girls or women lifting in the gym. She also ran a few times per week on the beach or the hilly trails near her home for 3 to 5 miles, sometimes up to 10 miles. At the time, she weighed only 93 pounds and had lower back pain, she says, and thought building up her muscles would help. She was already strong for her size. "I was the only girl in class to be able to do Body-weight dips," she recalls.

Within that first year of training, Jill put on a significant amount of muscle and looked lean, feminine, and healthy. "I noticed that exercise helped with my depression, lifted a fog, and gave me the ability to control the appearance of my physique," she says. "Weightlifting made me feel powerful and gave me control of at least a couple variables in my life."

She continued to train her Body with weights over the years, even during her pregnancy with twins. "Lifting became therapy for me," she says. "It was as habitual as brushing my teeth or combing my hair."

After the sudden death of her father in 2016, Jill took her bodybuilding hobby to the next level and decided to participate in figure competitions. "I'm an introvert who prefers being at home with a good book rather than prancing nearly naked on stage in front of judges and spectators," she says. "But reflecting on what I learned from my dad, I realized that I needed to step out of my box and start doing things that made me uncomfortable so that I could become a better person for myself and for others. Within the last several years, I have learned so much that I can share with my clients to help them grow, heal, and encourage them to conquer their goals."

Despite her apprehensions, she did very well, immediately receiving the coveted "pro card" and advancing to compete for the International Federation of Bodybuilding and Fitness (IFBB), the largest, most recognized bodybuilding organization in the world. Once at the pro level, competitors are able to earn money from the organization if they place in the top three in the open division. At a competition in 2020, Jill won the masters division (age 40 and over) and placed in the top five in the all-ages division, moving one step closer to qualifying for Figure Olympia, the most prestigious figure competition in the US.

Without bodybuilding and figure competitions, Jill says, she would not have learned so much about the Body and how to support it, to help it achieve demands that she places on it. "We can all read books and take classes, but until we live it, face challenges, and learn how to fix issues, we will not be completely thorough."

Bodybuilding is a unique physical activity, quintessential in its focus on the Body. It requires training muscles to acquire a specific and symmetrical appearance, with such precise definition that they can be seen as if there were no skin covering them. It takes an almost monastic approach as part athlete and part sculptor. Such precision can be meditative.

"As a bodybuilder, I think about my Body most of the time, even when I'm not competing," Jill says. "Some may view that as being consumed or even superficial, but I see it differently. Certainly, I want to look good, healthy, and youthful—we all want that—but it's more than that for me. The Body talks to us and gives us clues to its needs. If you listen or look, you can fix or adjust things before they lead to something detrimental."

What once was a means for Jill to strengthen and sculpt her Body has turned into a way to strengthen her Mind and spirit. "Bodybuilding has molded me as a person and has helped me accept myself," she says. "It has helped me learn to control my Mind and responses and push me out of my comfort zone to grow. I continue to push through things when they are difficult or when I don't feel like doing them. It has taught me that we have so much power within ourselves if we can learn how to harness that power in our Minds. Getting control of the Body is huge."

—⁓—

"Why do peacocks have ornate feathers?" I asked my eighth-grade teacher on a school field trip to the zoo.

"To attract the female peacocks," she responded.

Her answer was pretty close. Charles Darwin, whose theory of natural selection became the fundamental tenet of evolution—traits or behaviors that increase a species' fitness survive, while traits or behaviors that do not increase a species' fitness do not survive—also believed that characteristics evolve not just because they confer some kind of environmental advantage (i.e., they increase a species' "fitness"), but also because they confer a reproductive advantage. Darwin called this *sexual selection*. In other words, the peacock's fancy feathers evolved to ensure its reproductive success by providing a competitive advantage to attract peahens. As Darwin wrote, "Sexual selection depends, not on a struggle for existence, but on a struggle between the males for possession of the females; the result is not death to the unsuccessful competitor, but few or no offspring." Thus, while natural selection favors traits or behaviors that increase a species' fitness, sexual selection benefits mating. Darwin elaborates in *On the Origin of Species*:

Thus it is, as I believe, that when the males and females of any animal have the same general habits of life, but differ in structure, colour, or ornament, such differences have been mainly caused by sexual selection; that is, individual males have had, in successive generations, some slight advantage over other males, in their weapons, means of defence, or charms; and have transmitted these advantages to their male offspring.

As the handsome peacock struts his Body to attract the peahens, so too does the handsome man to attract the woman. Ever notice that many women love athletes? The girl who gets the high school football quarterback is often the envy of her friends. Sexual selection is the evolutionary reason for why girls want to date the quarterback.

In humans, as well as in many other animals, the attractiveness of one's Body is often linked to physical fitness, with a strong correlation between males' physical fitness and females' perception of the attractiveness of the male Body.[1] Indeed, a key function of the attractiveness of males' bodies is to *signal* their physical fitness, which was a highly desirable characteristic for mating in ancestral times. A female's ability to perceive physically fit males as attractive is an evolved adaptation. While we often like to think that what a person looks like is his or her least important quality, that what's on the inside is what really matters, the physical nature of our existence and its basis for sexual selection proves that what's on the outside matters, too. Peacocks could have black feathers; their feathers are colorful for a reason.

Throughout the longest time of human history, survival strongly depended on physical fitness, as our ancestors hunted for food and cared for themselves and their families. Physically fit males were better prepared for the violence that existed among competing males. They could be more physically aggressive to elevate their own status, co-opt others' resources, and protect their mates and their children against violence. Physically fit males would have passed on this physically fit advantage to their off-spring, as survival of the fittest dominated ancestral life.

Since superior athletic performance suggests a more fit mate and thus greater reproductive success, women perceive a good athlete as more attractive. A study at the University of Zurich in Switzerland found that cyclists who placed higher in the Tour de France were rated more attractive than cyclists who placed lower, and, interestingly, the preference for better cyclists was strongest in women not using a hormonal contraceptive.[2] The study also found that even heterosexual men rated the better male cyclists as more attractive, although the association wasn't as strong as when women were doing the rating. This preference for athletic performance works the other way, too, with men often finding female athletes to be more sexually attractive than nonathletes and even than lower-performing athletes.[3] Other research has shown that both women and men perceive athletes on teams and in individual sports as being more competitive, less lazy, and healthier than nonathletes, which increases their sexual selection.

Exercise enhances the Body's appearance, providing a competitive advantage to attract a sexual partner. But making yourself more physically attractive to the man or woman you meet in a bar, at the gym, or on a dating app is only part of the story. Daily exercise increases your physical fitness, enhancing your health and enabling you to thrive as an individual, and increases our collective Darwinian fitness, enhancing our sexual selection and enabling us to thrive as a species.

In his 2005 commencement speech at Kenyon College, novelist David Foster Wallace told the story of two young fish that were swimming upstream when another older fish approached them swimming the other way. "Hi, guys," said the older fish. "How's the water?"

As the two young fish continued swimming, one turned to the other and said, "What the hell is water?"

While the Body is the most inescapable and permanent aspect of our lives, like the water that surrounds the fish, we're not always aware of it. It is often absent from our Mind, as we attend to and focus on other things. But the Body is part of every nanosecond of every day of our lives.

My acute awareness of and interest in the human Body may have begun when I accidentally slammed a dresser drawer on my crown jewels when I was 6 years old. Ouch. My mother was so worried that the little accident would prevent me from ever having kids that she rushed me to the nearest emergency room to get them checked out. Of course, 6 years of age is still several years away from being able to test their effectiveness for producing offspring. Nonetheless, she had to be sure.

Or perhaps my interest began when I was 8 years old, when the left ventricle of my father's heart suffered so much damage from a heart attack that he never came out of the hospital. He was 51. I had lost my father, whose long walking strides on the Brooklyn, New York, sidewalks caused me to run to keep up.

Or perhaps it began when I was 11 years old, running one lap around a 400-meter track as fast as I could that started my life as a runner, enraptured by the complete and utter freedom of all-out physical effort. For as long as I can remember, I have been very high on the kinesthetics scale, the little collision between my crown jewels and the dresser drawer notwithstanding. Kinesthetics, from the Greek word *kinein*, "to move," is the perception of one's Body movements through space. I discovered early on that training the Body increases awareness of our physical being and improves kinesthetics.

Or perhaps it began when I was 13 years old, when I raised my chin above a wall-mounted bar in my school's gym twenty-four times in eighth grade to break my middle school chin-up record. I still have the certificate of achievement from the school's principal proudly displayed on my wall. I still brag about the accomplishment to others. It doesn't matter that it was so many years ago or that some tough kid has probably come along since to break my record. At the time, I had the strongest biceps and forearms in middle school. I used chin-ups to show off to girls. My mother even bought a chin-up bar and attached it to my bedroom doorframe so I could train at home. I did chin-ups every day.

Regardless of exactly when my interest in the human Body began, it has captivated me for a long time.

And I'm not the only one. The bodily nature of our existence, with its approximately 7 octillion atoms (that's a 7 followed by twenty-seven zeros) and 30 trillion cells (that's a 3 followed by thirteen zeros), has for long been a subject that has interested scientists. When one considers the interdisciplinary fields of biology, anatomy, zoology, biochemistry, biomechanics, physical therapy, psychology, exercise physiology, medicine, immunology, endocrinology, neurology, pharmacology, and public health, there is perhaps more research on the Body than on anything else ever researched. We are, collectively, fascinated by the animal Body, from the electrically charged cells of eels and catfish that help them navigate murky waters, to the biological compass of migratory birds that enables them to detect and be guided by Earth's magnetic fields on long-distance flights, to the acute sense of smell of wolves that enables them to detect other animals more than a mile away, to the collagenous tongues of chameleons that rapidly shoot out to one-and-a-half times their Body length to catch insects, and to the remarkable capacity of the human Brain to remember specific events, learn complex subjects like calculus, and create and articulate language.

The oldest documentation of a scientific study of the human Body during physical activity may be the classic book of seventeenth century scientist Giovanni Alphonso Borelli, *De Motu Animalium* (*Of Animal Motion*), in which he notes the relationships between leg length, stride rate, and running speed. The classic photography of Eadweard Muybridge at the end of the nineteenth century and beginning of the twentieth century in *Animals in Motion* and *The Human Figure in Motion* may have been the first attempt at photographing animal and human movement and is still referenced as the authority on walking and running mechanics. In the twentieth century, the most prominent researcher of locomotion may have been R. McNeill Alexander, PhD, of the University of Leeds in England, who combined zoology and physics to help elucidate the complexities of animal movement. Most recently, Dennis Bramble, PhD, of the University of Utah, and Daniel Lieberman, PhD, of Harvard University, have proposed through evolutionary research that long-distance running and walking were central to our evolutionary progress and shaped our anatomy, including our Brain.

The interesting contemporary research on robotics has shown that locomotion can be accomplished without sophisticated cognition (or, in the case of a robot, from a "controller" that acts like a Brain), but rather through exploiting the dynamics of the Body and its interaction with the environment.[4] When the Body of a robot is optimally designed, it can walk down an incline without any control from motors, sensors, and microprocessors—in other words, without a Brain. The robot's ability to walk down an incline is an outcome of the slope of the incline, gravity, and the mechanical features of the robot's Body, including its leg segment lengths, mass distribution, and foot shape.

It is impossible to separate human life, or the life of any other organism, from the physical Body in which it lives. Even without slamming your reproductive organ with a dresser drawer, we are reminded of this every day.

Every day, you must sleep many hours.

Every day, you must eat multiple times.

Every day, you must go to the bathroom several times.

Every day, you must cater to your physical needs to continue living.

Without sleep, food and drink, and going to the bathroom, your life ends. That's why it is such a strong urge to do these things. It is such a strong urge to take care of your Body.

Your earthly life begins with your Body and ends with your Body. From your first heartbeat to your last. It is virtually impossible to live without movement of the Body.

Since the *Tiktaalik* fish that wriggled its way out of the sea and propped itself up on land with its sturdy fins about 375 million years ago, life on land was off and running. Those fins slowly evolved into limbs over millions of years, as animals, including eventually humans, interacted with their new environments.

With those limbs, we crawl almost immediately after being born, then stand on two of them to walk shortly thereafter, and begin running soon after that. It doesn't take anyone to tell us to do it or teach us to do it. We do it automatically. We could have stopped with crawling. We could have stopped with walking. But we didn't. And we don't.

We run because we are animals, and running is what animals evolved to do. Running is essential to an animal's life. Animals run to hunt, they run because they're being hunted, they run to play, they run out of panic, and they even run to flirt with and show off to other members of their species. On school playgrounds across the world, human animals also show off their speed, as children race each other during recess.

Millions of years ago, hunting and gathering food and procreation were the initial reasons for humans living a physically active life. We ran, we made weapons and other products with our hands, and we had sexual intercourse, because that is what humans had to do to survive as individuals and as a species.

Throughout a long history, humans have had to depend on themselves whenever they wanted to go somewhere, and sometimes they wanted to go somewhere quickly. The hunter-gatherer lifestyle of our ancestors, which dominated human life until the Neolithic era (10,000 to 4,500 BC), required the ability to sustain a high level of aerobic physical activity, fundamentally affecting the development of human anatomy and physiology. Humans had to run, and by running, humans became animals that run. The Body is specifically made for running and the physical life. Had early humans stuck to walking, we would now be quite physically different. Our Body would not be what it is and would not function as it does.

Our heart never would have reached the maximum stroke volume of 200 milliliters of blood per beat, nor the maximum rate of 190 or more beats per minute that a trained young adult runner's heart can reach.

Our muscles never would have developed the 60,000 miles of capillaries that surround them, like intricate spiderwebs, to deliver oxygen.

Our Achilles tendon, which connects the heel bone to the calf muscle, never would have become a spring to store and return energy with every step.

Our lungs never would have developed such a thin wall over such an enormous area to become the perfect medium for oxygen and carbon dioxide gas exchange.

Our eccrine glands never would have developed into such efficient sweat producers that enable rapid evaporation and the ability to regulate Body temperature as our ancestors traversed very hot environments on foot.

Our foot's arch never would have become such an effective shock absorber, like an expertly engineered suspension bridge, capable of absorbing the shock of landing on the ground with many times our Body weight.

These evolutionary traits, together with bipedal gait, increases in Body and skull size, and the loss of Body hair, have had a large impact on present-day exercise capacity in humans.

Parallel to the macrochanges to the Body that occurred over the long term from evolution, microchanges to the Body occur over the short term throughout your life. Physical exercise in general, and muscle contraction in particular, cause many agitations inside your cells that disturb metabolic homeostasis. These agitations stir up your DNA to promote adaptive responses, including changes in messenger RNA and protein levels inside your Body.[5,6]

While you cannot change your *genotype*—the genetic makeup of your microscopic cells that lie deep within you and provide the code for who you are—training your Body has the remarkable ability to change your *phenotype*—the way those genes express themselves and interact with your environment to create your traits. Genes are constantly activated and inhibited—turned on and off—depending on the biochemical signals they receive from their environment. Through modifications to your DNA by the chemical processes of methylation, acetylation, and phosphorylation, genes become more responsive to signals in their environment, which regulates protein function, overall health, and the way you think and learn.[7]

In a clever experiment to isolate the effect of physical exercise on individuals' genes, scientists at the prestigious Karolinska Institute in Stockholm, Sweden, had twenty-three men and women cycle with one leg on a stationary bicycle at a moderate pace for 45 minutes four times per week for three months, while the other leg did not exercise. Before and after the experiment, the scientists administered a series of physical and medical tests, including a muscle biopsy.

Not surprisingly, the trained leg was more powerful than the untrained leg after three months, showing that the exercise program had resulted in physical improvements. But the DNA between legs was also different. Using genomic analysis, the scientists discovered that more than 5,000 sites on the genome of muscle cells from the trained leg showed significant changes in DNA methylation and gene expression, while the DNA of the untrained leg remained unchanged.

Physical exercise, especially when that exercise is repeated over and over and over again, such that it becomes a chronic state (i.e., training), is one of the most potent stimuli to change the Body. What's most impressive about exercise is the number of characteristics it changes and enhances and the number of conditions and diseases it either prevents, ameliorates, or delays. Exercise increases blood volume, the number of red blood cells, and hemoglobin, all of which increase your blood vessels' oxygen transport. Exercise creates a greater network of capillaries, which increases diffusion of oxygen into your muscles. Exercise makes your heart bigger, which enables it to pump more blood with each beat. Exercise increases the amount of fuel stored in your muscles, which improves your muscular endurance. Exercise increases the size and number of mitochondria and the number of enzymes contained within them, which increases your muscles' aerobic metabolic capacity. Exercise increases the size of your muscle fibers, which makes you stronger. Exercise increases the number of neurons and synapses in your Brain, which makes you smarter. Exercise strengthens your immune system, which means you'll get fewer colds and other infections. Exercise increases the activity of your parasympathetic nervous system, which slows your resting heart rate and reduces your blood pressure. Exercise increases good HDL cholesterol and reduces bad LDL cholesterol, which reduces the risk for cardiovascular disease. Exercise reduces Body fat, which also reduces the risk for cardiovascular disease and changes the way you look and the amount of space you take up in your environment. Exercise makes your cells more receptive to insulin, which maintains blood sugar levels and reduces the risk for diabetes. Exercise increases bone density, which reduces the risk of fractures as you age. Exercise increases testosterone in both men and women (although the effect of exercise on testosterone is much more pronounced in men), which has many physiological effects, and even increases libido and your response to sexual stimulation.[8]

Humans are so hardwired for a physical lifestyle that the absence of physical activity not only prevents these changes from occurring, it causes regression and atrophy of Body structures and functions, which reduces your Body's cardiac and physiological reserve and, consequently, its ability to cope with environmental stressors. This leaves the door wide open to many diseases and pathophysiological conditions, including obesity, heart disease, osteoporosis, and diabetes, and accelerates aging, with an earlier onset of frailty and a lower quality of life.[9,10]

That there is a cost to not being physically active should not come as a surprise, especially when we remember that humans are animals. No one would ever think of a lion as a sedentary animal. When you think of a lion, or even your pet German shepherd, you think of physical activity.

But we see ourselves as different from other animals, perhaps because they don't look or act like us.

Human attitudes toward other animals have a lot to do with physical and functional similarity. As with other humans, we like and relate more to other animals that we perceive are more like us, both in physical attributes and in behavior.[11] But even when compared to our nearest ancestors—chimpanzees and bonobos—we still see ourselves as different, as "non-animal." But we are much more similar than we want to admit; our DNA is 95 to 99 percent similar to that of chimpanzees.

Like other animals, humans live by a circadian rhythm that is dictated by light and dark. Throughout evolution, animals, including human animals, have exploited the light and dark patterns of day and night to feed or avoid being food. We are awake during the light hours of the day and we sleep during the dark hours of the night. Certain conditions that interrupt this pattern often cause problems. For example, individuals who work night shifts and world travelers who cross time zones often experience fatigue and have trouble adjusting to the unnatural patterns.

Given other animals' cognitive limitations that prevent them from being self-conscious of their physical appearance and aware of the health consequences of an inactive lifestyle, it is almost certain that other animals don't exercise with intentions similar to those of humans. While animals in the wild have been recorded engaging in what appears to be voluntary exercise, it is unknown what those animals' intentions are for doing so, or whether or not there are intentions at all.[12]

Perhaps other animals intuitively or instinctively know that improving fitness helps them chase or avoid being chased, or perhaps they exercise simply because it feels good. Many studies have shown that when a running wheel is placed in a mouse's cage, the mouse runs on the wheel. It's hard to imagine that the mouse runs for the intention of looking good in its jeans, lowering its cholesterol, or training for a marathon. It's likely that the mouse runs because running is the mouse's instinct.

In modern times, the daily life of many animals is still physically intense enough to reach an effective level of fitness to thrive in their environments. But this is no longer true for humans. Unlike a mouse, a shark, or an eagle, humans, for the most part, cannot maintain such an effective fitness level solely from the activities of daily modern living. Our contemporary sedentary lifestyle necessitates that specific time be set aside for exercise to maintain physical fitness—of individuals and of the species.

Today, we don't run as much as our ancestors did. We don't make things with our hands. We don't hunt and chase other animals for food. We have lost our animal ways. The energy expenditure attributed to the physical activity of today's office worker is only one quarter that of our ancestor *Homo erectus* 1.7 million years ago.[13] But since cultural changes occur faster than genetic evolution, our genes remain adapted for the conditions that existed during their selection.[14,15] In other words, the Body wants to be used, wants to be trained, wants to be fit. Apart from biology, physical activity is deep in our social history. The ancient Greeks, who gave us the first fitness centers (large open areas called *gymnasiums*), competitive sport, and the Olympic Games, worshipped the Body. Running was a highly regarded physical trait. Most modern runners are familiar with the legendary run of the Greek messenger Pheidippides from the battleground of Marathon to the marketplace in Athens to announce the Greeks' war victory over the Persians. It is from the starting point of his run in Greece that we get the name of the race that millions of people around the world run each year. We run and engage in other forms of exercise not just because it is good for us biologically, but also to explore our outer spaces and the inner space within the individual self. What drives us to be physically active is the need to feel human. Because the human experience is physical.

Jon picked up the Coca-Cola can that sat next to his computer, revealing a water ring mark on the thick mahogany desk. After taking a sip, he placed the can back on the ring and paused to take a deep breath, inhaling the stiff office air.

"It's been a long time since I thought of my life as being so physical," Jon said.

"I'm afraid few people ever think of their life that way," I responded. "People tend to focus on their Mind rather than on their Body, as if the Mind is the most sacred part of them, as if the Mind is in control.

"Even though Body, Brain, and Mind are often in conflict, Jon, the Body must always be the boss," I said. "Because the Body is the vehicle you use to navigate life. You are an animal. An attorney is simply what you have chosen to do for your financial success so you can pay your bills. But you were born an animal. You were not born an attorney.

"Remember what it was like when you were running 90 miles per week? You were an athlete. Your Body was the boss. You were able to complete college and law school while running 90 miles per week.

"And you only failed a few exams," I joked.

"I remember," Jon replied with a laugh.

"Why did you run that much, Jon?" I asked. Being a lifelong runner myself, I knew his answer, but I wanted him to say it out loud.

Jon turned away to stare out the window before responding, as if to look outside of himself to remember the answer. "I enjoyed seeing my Body improve and get faster," he replied. "I enjoyed listening to my Body while I ran. I enjoyed the soulful feeling I got after a hard effort."

"Interesting," I replied. "You see how your reasons for running are connected to your Body?" I asked.

Jon nodded. "Yes," he said, as if he had just learned something.

"Most people go through every day of their lives without exerting any physical effort, without using the Body to its capacity. But physical activity, which enabled our ancient ancestors to adapt to and succeed in their environments, is part of human instinct. It is *instinctual* to be physically active. Throughout evolutionary history, the Body has always led the way.

"Because so much of the human life experience is embodied, people's perceptions of their physical attributes and competencies dictate much of their lives.

"When my mother was in the hospital during the final two weeks of her life, in pain from bone cancer, she rhetorically asked me, 'What kind of life is this?' Unable to get out of bed and walk on her own, she was ready to give up on life. She was ready to die. When our physical capabilities diminish, we lose a central part of our identity. We lose a central part of life.

"Running makes you a better attorney, Jon, and a better father and a better husband, because it makes you a better human. While it oftentimes may seem selfish to those around you, because working out takes time from things others may want you to immediately do for them, the benefits of working out accrue not only to yourself, but also to those around you in a wide range of ways, positively affecting both your professional and personal life.

"Like the *Tiktaalik* fish that left the water to come to land 375 million years ago, acting with the Body precedes knowing. The *Tiktaalik* fish didn't *know* that it could survive on land; it *acted* out of instinct, and the Brain caught up so that it could survive.

"Survival of the fittest.

"But the rewards of working out go far beyond physical fitness.

"Because when you train your Body, you change your Brain."

CHAPTER TWO

Brain

I'M FEELING GOOD NOW, AND
I'M GOING TO STICK WITH THAT

WALKING DOWN HAIGHT STREET IN SAN FRANCISCO, YOU COME across a small art studio with a 1960s-looking storefront, nestled among other 1960s-looking shops in the well-known hippie district of Haight-Ashbury. Inside the studio, an African American man with a gray goatee and a beanie sits on a stool and paints on a canvas. His artwork, much of which depicts scenes of San Francisco, adorns the walls.

Ronnie Goodman was a self-taught artist in San Francisco. Before his death in 2020 at 60 years of age, he had been painting nearly all his life. His art, he said, was inspired by the beauty and diversity of San Francisco, balanced with the struggles of human despair.

"With my brush, I try to capture these raw emotions in painted images of the city," he told me, five years before he died. "I have a story to tell. I think I have a lot to say. It's very hard to make a living as an artist. The most important thing is that I don't give up."

When Ronnie Goodman wasn't painting, he ran. He ran up to 50 miles per week on the streets of San Francisco, often wearing a Tamalpa Racing singlet from the local Tamalpa Runners running club. He ran many half-marathons, including the San Francisco Half-Marathon in July 2014, which he ran for his birthday. He even ran the famous Dipsea Trail Race in Marin County, California, the oldest trail race in America.

If you had the chance to talk to Ronnie Goodman about his experiences of being a runner, it wouldn't have taken long to discover that his running and painting were intertwined. He spoke from his heart, yet was often nonchalant about things, brushing them off as if nothing special.

"Running helps inspire me as an artist," he said. "When I get stuck creating a piece of work, running helps me step back from the canvas and put ideas together. I can look at the canvas in my imagination."

Ronnie Goodman knew much of the human despair he painted about in the art studio on Haight Street. Experiencing depression after his mother passed away, he tried to self-medicate with drugs, using marijuana, heroin, and cocaine. He spent eight years in San Quentin Prison for burglary. He was homeless for twenty years. He had four kids, one of whom was stabbed to death. His ex-wife didn't want anything to do with him when he became a drug addict. "Once you get into drugs, you lose everything," he said.

Sober for the last seventeen years of his life, Ronnie lived a pretty simple life on the streets in San Francisco. He painted, and he ran. Even without having much to his name, he still gave back to the community that had supported his painting and running. He sold his prints, posters, greeting cards, and T-shirts in the art studio and on his website. He managed the studio in exchange for painting in it. He donated his artwork to churches. And he fundraised for Hospitality House, an organization that provides programs for San Francisco's homeless community.

Ronnie had been running on and off since elementary school. He was competitive in middle school, but didn't get serious about running until much later in life, ironically when he was in prison.

It was there that he met a volunteer named Frank, who started the 1,000 Miles Running Club at the prison. Ronnie joined so that he could do something healthy for himself.

While in prison, Ronnie ran four times per week for an hour to an hour and a half. Around a courtyard. He even ran four marathons in prison—105 laps around a quarter-mile track.

"Running gets you into a meditative mode," he said, slowly, as if he were meditating within his words. "It makes you see things differently. If I'm going through something that might have happened the day before that made me feel depressed, I put on my shoes and run, and it's like, 'Oh, it's a wrap; it's over with. I just ran, I feel good. I don't need to stick to those feelings that made me feel bad. I'm feeling good now, and I'm going to stick with that.'"

When I asked the former drug addict and ex-con how he ran being homeless, he said, "I just do." There's little more to that answer.

When asked *why* he runs, I got an answer that had *a lot* more to it. "When I'm running, I feel like I'm not there. I feel like I'm somewhere else. I feel like I'm inside of myself. It's like this spiritual moment that I'm just running and running. I might run for 2 hours, and I'm a free person for those 2 hours."

On the other side of the prison cell, Ronnie sometimes ran with his friend Frank, the prison volunteer who started the 1,000 Miles Running Club. But he usually ran alone, using his runs to imagine and create the art that he painted later that day.

Some would have looked at Ronnie Goodman and felt sorry for him, having died a homeless person, alone, in his encampment in the Mission District of San Francisco. But he didn't feel sorry for himself. Quite the contrary. In many ways, he turned his life around, and he lived the life that he wanted to live, painting and running and giving back to the community with his art.

I finished my conversation with Ronnie by asking him what he wanted people to know about him.

"I just want people to know I'm an artist and a runner. It makes me feel alive."

⁓

Lorenza Colzato, PhD, is an Italian cognitive psychologist at the Institute for Psychological Research and Leiden Institute for Brain and Cognition at Leiden University in the Netherlands. Her research focuses on the ways that thinking and creativity are shaped, including the effects of exercise.

Through her research, Colzato has found that people perform better on creative-thinking tests following a bout of aerobic exercise compared to when the tests are taken without exercising first.[1] She has also found that people who exercise score higher on creative-thinking tests than people who don't exercise. However, exercise only positively affected creative thinking in the individuals who were used to exercising.

Colzato's research suggests that if individuals are not used to exercising, the mental effort that goes into the exercise itself may detract from the ability to think creatively after the workout is over, as if the workout itself is exhausting mentally as well as physically. Other research has also shown that physically fit individuals are better able than unfit individuals to perform cognitive tasks during and after exercise, perhaps because of the direct effect exercise has on cognition or because of the positive view that fit people have toward exercise and the consequent expectation that exercise will improve their mood and mental clarity.[2]

Exercise unlocks your ability to think creatively, but *only if your Body is used to being active.*

I often come up with creative ideas while running. The rhythm of running enables those ideas to come to the surface; they are much more difficult to come up with when I'm sitting at my desk and concentrating on them.

While creativity is one of the most sought-after mental processes, it is perhaps the least understood. Science has linked creativity to mood, with positive moods generally improving creativity. A number of studies have shown that even a single session of aerobic exercise significantly enhances mood and creative thinking,[3] although it appears that the enhanced ability to think creatively is independent of any changes in mood, suggesting that creativity is not just a matter of mood.[4]

Research has also shown that exercise throughout life improves cognition and fluid intelligence, including problem-solving ability, memory, learning, and pattern recognition.[5,6,7] And in both elementary and high school, physical activity improves cognition, learning, and academic performance, even when the time spent being physically active decreases the time spent in the classroom or studying.[8,9] Training the Body indeed has cognitive consequences. Researchers in the field of education have argued that teaching and learning should not focus purely on the Brain to the exclusion of the Body, and that teachers often fail to consider the role that the Body plays in the cognitive skills they teach, instead treating those skills as being independent from the Body.[10,11]

The exercise-mediated improvements in cognitive function are even more observable as you age. Physical activity triggers molecular and cellular changes in the Brain, sustains cerebral blood low, increases nutrient supply to the Brain, and facilitates neurotransmitter metabolism, all of which help you to think better. There is considerable evidence that a lack of physical activity in the elderly is a risk factor for poor cognitive functioning. It seems that if you want to remain mentally sharp as you age, you had better exercise.

Exercise has such an effect on cognition that it even affects us before we're born. Research has shown that when mothers exercise while they're pregnant, their children's academic performance is superior to that of children whose mothers didn't exercise during pregnancy.[12,13] And in other animals, many laboratory studies have shown that mothers who are either forced to exercise or exercise voluntarily during pregnancy produce offspring that have more neurons and proteins in their Brains, greater long-term Brain plasticity, and show improved learning and memory throughout their lives compared to offspring whose mothers don't exercise when pregnant.[14]

Why does training the Body enhance creativity and cognition? To answer this question, we need to understand what's happening when we're being creative and when we're thinking, and for that we need to look beyond our cardiovascular and muscular systems.

We need to look inside the Brain.

Perhaps the most significant evolutionary advance to create the modern human is the central nervous system. The primitive hormonal pathways that linked features of the environment to responses of organisms evolved into actual physical pathways in the Brain, with neurons, axons, dendrites, and neurotransmitters, creating a modern-day human Brain that is the most complex system known in the universe. This intricate system enables you to think about things in a way that other animals cannot. It is the source of human creativity. It enables you to mix food ingredients to cook a delicious dinner, to read and understand Shakespeare, and to drive a car at 60 miles per hour, and it enables me to put thousands of words together to write this book.

The evolution of the Brain's physical structures caused it to grow, in evolutionary timelines, rather quickly, from 600 grams as *Homo habilis* 2 million years ago, to 850 to 1,200 grams as *Homo erectus* 1.5 million to 130,000 years ago, to 1,400 grams as *Homo sapiens*, first showing up 130,000 years ago.[15,16] The human cerebellum, which is responsible for coordinating voluntary physical movements and for balance, coordination, and posture, is three times larger than that of an ape.[17] In addition to the approximately 86 billion neurons inside your Brain, half a million motor neurons and 10 million sensory neurons all over your Body, which are responsible for movement and sensory perceptions, communicate so closely with your Brain that they, too, are virtually part of it.

Your Brain "reads" sensory signals generated by the Body, which, through its interaction with its environment, is responsible for the representations of the world around you. That reading, which is translated into cognition, comes second, and is in the service of the physical Body. Your movements enable your Brain to perceive change, which then enables your Brain to plan your subsequent movements and actions. This is why toddlers who are slow to get on their feet to move around their environment, as well as children who are late in achieving other developmental motor markers, are at a high risk for cognitive impairment.[18] The Brain is subservient to motor development, with its neural systems contributing to your cognition later in life.

But since the Brain also controls your Body's movements, the relationship between the Body and the Brain is reciprocal and interdependent: Abnormal cognition impairs movement and abnormal movement impairs cognition. For example, children with ADHD, dyslexia, and autism commonly have motor coordination problems and movement deficits.[19] When genetic or environmental perturbations affect the Body's ability to move or the Brain's ability to think, both the Body and the Brain are often affected.

While you may not always be conscious of it, your Brain is constantly sensing both the external and internal states of your Body through two processes called *exteroception* and *interoception*. Through mechanoreceptors and proprioceptors in your skin to sensory and neural pathways originating from internal organs and physiological systems, exteroception and interoception are central to everything you are and do, from your movements and thoughts to your emotions and your sense of self. They enable you to answer the question, "How do you feel today?"

Exteroception is sensitivity to stimuli originating outside your Body and enables you to successfully interact with your environment. You see, hear, smell, taste, and touch the world around you. Exteroception is why you remove your hand from a hot stove (and why you don't put your hand on a hot stove in the first place).

Interoception is sensitivity to stimuli originating inside your Body. For example, your Brain senses when your Body needs energy (e.g., when blood glucose is low), and decides to eat based on its sensory perception. (Interoception is also why it's harder to think and to exercise when you're hungry. When there's a metabolic deficit, like low blood glucose, and your Body needs energy, your Brain reduces its spending on things that are expensive, such as learning new information and physical movement.) Beyond satisfying physical urges, interoception enables you to know you're scared or anxious or happy.

Cognition cannot be understood without understanding the state of the Body that contributes to that cognition. Thoughts are not driving feelings; rather, feelings (from the Body) are driving thoughts. The Body is thus crucial for the Brain's perception. As the Brain perceives what is going on outside and inside the Body, it efficiently ensures resources for the Body's physiological systems so that it can grow, survive, thrive, and reproduce.[20]

You probably don't recognize his name, but Raymond Damadian has had a significant impact on understanding how you think. Damadian, an American physician of Armenian descent, earned a bachelor's degree in mathematics from the University of Wisconsin–Madison in 1956 and an MD degree from the Albert Einstein College of Medicine in New York in 1960. An eclectic fellow, he studied the violin at the famous Juilliard School for eight years and was a good enough tennis player in his youth that he played in Junior Davis Cup tennis tournaments.

Using nuclear magnetic resonance, Damadian was one of the first people to notice differences in the molecular structure between normal and diseased tissue. In 1977, he invented a way to detect the distinctive radio frequencies from a spot the size of a pea within the living human Body. Damadian's invention garnered him the National Medal of Technology by the president of the United States and an induction into the National Inventors Hall of Fame. There's a good chance you have used his machine yourself. His MRI scanning device is in practically every hospital and medical clinic in the world, diagnosing everything from a stress fracture of a bone to a stroke in the Brain. MRI can give us a clear picture of what's going on in the Brain, from structural abnormalities to blood flow and tumors to degeneration.

Advancing Damadian's invention was Japanese biophysicist and neuroscientist Seiji Ogawa, whose discovery of the functional MRI technique (fMRI) enables scientists to see what's going on in the Brain during specific activities. Ogawa determined that the changes in blood oxygen levels in the Brain cause its MRI to change. Since oxygen is used by active neurons, fMRI can distinguish neurons that are functionally active from those that are less active or inactive, giving scientists and doctors insight into the Brain's functional activity.

Using fMRI, scientists can tell which parts of your Brain are active when you do puzzles, when you look at facial expressions to determine and empathize with someone's feelings, and even when you exercise.

For this latter insight, scientists at the University of Campinas in São Paulo, Brazil, and the University of Cape Town in Cape Town, South Africa, used fMRI to compare Brain activity at different levels of perceived exertion while individuals cycled on a stationary bicycle.[21] The exercise session was designed as an interval workout—six 2-minute reps of cycling with 16-second rest periods between reps—so that Brain activity between exercise and rest periods and between easier and harder exercise reps could be compared.

When cycling, certain parts of the Brain—the cerebellar vermis and precentral and postcentral gyrus, which are involved in controlling Body posture and motor activity—were active compared to during the rest periods. As the workout became physically difficult and perceived exertion increased, other areas of the Brain—the posterior cingulate gyrus and precuneus, which are involved in responses to pain, motivation, episodic memory retrieval, and introspection—became more active.

Functional MRI research has shown that certain parts of the Brain are also more active—with greater blood flow and increased functional connectivity—following aerobic exercise. Functional connectivity—areas of the Brain that are functionally connected despite not being physically connected—is a correlational relationship between regionally distinct areas of the Brain that are synchronized in time through fluctuations of activity. It is measured using blood oxygenation level–dependent signals in the Brain during resting conditions.

While a single workout transiently increases functional connectivity, chronic physical training causes permanent changes. When fMRI is used to compare functional connectivity between trained distance runners and age-matched sedentary individuals, clear differences are found in functional connectivity.[22] Time spent running and level of aerobic fitness are both associated with greater functional connectivity in networks that are linked to executive function and motor control.

To find out if functional connectivity depends on the intensity of exercise, scientists at the University Hospital Bonn in Bonn, Germany, used fMRI to measure functional connectivity in three different Brain networks in twenty-five physically active males following 30 minutes of low-intensity (35 percent below lactate threshold) and high-intensity (20 percent above lactate threshold) treadmill running on separate days.[23] They found that functional connectivity increased following low-intensity exercise in the frontoparietal network, which is responsible for sustained attention, complex problem-solving, working memory, and mood. Functional connectivity also increased following low-intensity exercise and decreased following high-intensity exercise in the sensorimotor network, which is responsible for performing and coordinating motor tasks. Finally, functional connectivity increased following high-intensity exercise and decreased following low-intensity exercise in the affective and reward network, which is responsible for self-awareness through the integration of sensory, emotional, and cognitive information.

━ ━

For many years before MRI, the human Brain was thought to never change after birth. "There's the old way of viewing the older adult Brain, which is viewing the Brain like a rock," says Kirk Erickson, PhD, professor of psychology at the University of Pittsburgh. "As we get older, the rock hardens, and your Brain hardens, and, if you damage or chip the rock, you're not going to recover. It's less flexible. But in recent years, we know that's not the case. We can alter the functioning of the Brain. This type of decline is not inevitable."

Erickson's research focuses on how cognition and the structure and function of the Brain change across the lifespan. He is one of only a few scientists who have made fundamental discoveries relating exercise to Brain growth and the preservation of cognition as humans age. Some of his research has focused on N-acetylaspartate (NAA), the second most abundant amino acid in the Brain, found predominantly in the cell bodies of neurons. It exists exclusively in neural tissue and is essential for normal Brain function. The amount of NAA in the Brain is associated with obesity, type 2 diabetes, and cognitive dysfunction in neuro-degenerative diseases.

To assess whether neuronal viability is a mechanism by which physical fitness enhances cognition in the elderly, Erickson and his colleagues used magnetic resonance spectroscopy to measure the level of NAA in the frontal cortex of 137 healthy, older men and women, along with their aerobic fitness.[24] They found that older age was associated with less NAA in the frontal cortex of the Brain, while greater aerobic fitness was associated with more NAA in the Brain, offsetting the age-related decline in NAA. They also found a positive correlation between the amount of NAA in the Brain and both cardiovascular fitness and working memory. "Higher aerobic fitness levels ameliorate an age-related decline in NAA concentrations in the frontal cortex," Erickson says, "and higher NAA concentrations mediate the association between aerobic fitness and working memory span."

Erickson's research has revealed that, like the Brains of younger individuals, the Brains of older individuals are capable of change. Specifically, age-related patterns of deterioration can be reversed, with such reversal significantly improving cognition and Brain function in older adults.

It's an interesting field of science called *neuroplasticity*—the flexibility of the Brain to change, adapt to different situations, and improve its functioning.

And the biggest thing that makes the Brain change?

Exercise.

Like your muscles, your Brain senses and adapts to exercise. From childhood to old age, exercise is good for your Brain, your cognitive capabilities, and your mood.[25,26] A robust finding of scientific research is that exercise and physical fitness positively affect Brain health in seniors and retard the age-related decline in cognitive function, with both aerobic and resistance exercise improving cognitive function in older adults.[27-31]

As we age, most notably past 60 years, we experience many biological changes in our Brains, including the shrinkage of neurons, the reduction in the branching of dendrites of neurons (which reduces the number of synapses), loss of myelination (which reduces the speed of signal transmission along a neuron), decreases in neurotransmitters, and reduction in cerebral blood flow. All these changes reduce the amount and speed of communication between neurons in your Brain. And that means you can't remember where you parked your car in the stadium parking lot when the baseball game is over. But getting and staying fit can help you find your car.

Your Brain structure is related to your muscle structure. As it does with skeletal muscles and cardiac muscle, exercise causes structural and functional changes in your Brain.[32] These changes may have conferred an evolutionary advantage given the evidence that, in nonhuman mammals, there is a positive correlation between maximum aerobic exercise capacity and Brain size.[33] In humans, exercise increases the volume of multiple regions of the Brain, including the frontal lobe, temporal lobe, parietal lobe, and hippocampus, and prevents the atrophy that often accompanies aging. Specifically, two parts of your Brain are affected the most by exercise—the prefrontal cortex and the hippocampus.

The prefrontal cortex, the part of the cerebral cortex that covers the front part of your Brain's frontal lobe, is responsible for executive functions, such as personality expression, decision-making, planning complex cognitive behavior, and moderating social behavior. In short, the prefrontal cortex orchestrates your Mind and actions in accordance with your goals.

The hippocampus, which sits under the cerebral cortex in your Brain's medial temporal lobe, is critically important for long-term memory, spatial navigation and memory (the ability to remember an object's location relative to other objects in its environment), and the regulation of emotions.

In both younger and older adults, higher levels of fitness are associated with a larger Brain volume, specifically of the prefrontal cortex and hippocampus.[34] Conversely, an inactive daily life is a risk factor for Brain atrophy, specifically of the frontal lobe—the part of your Brain responsible for emotions, problem-solving, reasoning, and planning. Specifically, the frontal lobe affects your ability to recognize future consequences resulting from current actions, the choice between good and bad actions, the suppression of socially unacceptable responses, and your ability to determine similarities and differences between things or events. All these factors are negatively affected by lack of exercise as you age and positively affected by staying or becoming active. Exercise also facilitates the interaction between the frontal lobe's prefrontal cortex and the amygdala. The prefrontal cortex helps dampen the amygdala's fear and anxiety signals. With fewer constraints from fear and anxiety, you can think more clearly and freely.

If you were to view a slice of your Brain, you would see two types of tissue—gray matter, which consists of neuron cell bodies, dendrites, nerve fibers, synapses, and capillaries; and white matter, which consists of nerve fibers covered by myelin, an insulation of fatty tissue that increases the speed of electrical nerve signals. Gray matter includes regions of the Brain involved in muscle control, seeing and hearing, memory, emotions, speech, decision-making, and self-control. White matter modulates the distribution of nerve signals so that different regions of your Brain can communicate with each other. Think of gray matter as multiple computers and white matter as the electrical cables that transmit signals between them.

Like skeletal muscles, gray matter volume, along with total Brain volume, atrophies with age.[35] Loss of skeletal muscle from aging is actually a risk factor for Brain atrophy.[36] The good news is that physical activity suppresses the Brain atrophy induced by aging and increases gray matter and retains Brain volume, specifically of the prefrontal cortex and hippocampus, areas of the Brain that tend to decline earlier in adulthood and that involve executive functions and memory.[37] Physical activity also increases the amount of gray matter in late adulthood, making exercise an effective prevention for cognitive impairment and other behavioral problems associated with Brain atrophy.[38]

Physical activity also increases white matter. Interestingly, the speed at which a person can walk, and even the strength of one's grip, is significantly related to the volume of white matter.[39] In one study, scientists at Wake Forest University's School of Medicine administered a battery of cognitive tests to 2,349 well-functioning adults aged 70 to 79 years old over a three-year period and measured their speed of walking.[40] They found a significant relationship between cognition and the decline in walking speed. For every one-standard-deviation-lower performance on each cognitive test, there was a greater decline in walking speed. Another study on 675 older adults also found that cognition was strongly related to walking speed, with slower walkers performing worse on cognition tests, faster walkers performing better on cognition tests, and the intermediate-speed walkers performing in the middle.[41] Reduced cognitive function is associated with a subsequent decline in physical performance in late life. Older individuals who can walk at a faster speed have more white matter, better cognition, and a less aged Brain.

You have approximately 86 billion neurons in your Brain.[42,43] That's a lot of neurons (albeit less than the 100 billion that scientists used to think the Brain had before more recent precise counts have been made). Think about that for a second. That's more than twelve times the number of people on Earth. All inside your head. For comparison, our nearest ancestor, the chimpanzee, has 28 billion neurons, while an ant has just 250,000 neurons.

The more neurons in the Brain, regardless of Brain or Body size, the better a species performs a given task. Although chimpanzees are very smart, they can't hit an Aroldis Chapman fastball or beat world champion Garry Kasparov at a game of chess.

For a long time, the number of neurons in the Brain was thought to be a fixed number based on what you're born with. In his 1928 book, *Degeneration and Regeneration of the Nervous System*, Santiago Ramón y Cajal, the father of modern neuroscience, wrote, "In the adult centers, the nerve paths are something fixed, ended, and immutable. Everything may die, nothing may be regenerated."[44]

But that's not the way it is.

If increasing the volume of your Brain isn't enough to make you more creative, exercise does something even more spectacular to your Brain. It causes the formation of new neurons, called *neurogenesis*.[45–50] Previously thought to occur only in the developing Brain of a fetus and newborn, it's now accepted that those 86 billion neurons that you were born with can increase throughout your life. The existence of neurogenesis in adult mammals, first discovered in 1962 by biologist Joseph Altman in the Brains of rats, has provided much insight into the adaptability of the Brain.[51,52] In 1998, using postmortem tissue from the hippocampus and the subventricular zone of the caudate nucleus in the Brains of cancer patients, neuroscientist Peter Eriksson documented the occurrence of neurogenesis in humans and that the proliferation of the new Brain cells depends on environmental stimuli.[53]

Neurogenesis means that more neurons communicate with each other in your Brain. All that communication fosters what scientists call *divergent thinking*—thinking outside the box. "Exercise can influence both the structure of the Brain as well as its functional capacity," says Brian Christie, PhD, professor of medicine and neuroscience at the University of Victoria in British Columbia, Canada, whose research examines the biological processes underlying learning and memory in the mammalian Brain.

The hippocampus is the primary part of the Brain where neurogenesis occurs and is most influenced by exercise. When you try a new exercise or learn a new physical movement, the change in your Brain is temporary. But as you practice the exercise or movement, day in, day out, you cement that change, and it becomes a permanent part of your Brain's structure.

Interestingly, the hippocampus is one of the first regions of the Brain to suffer damage in patients with Alzheimer's disease. The hippocampus also contains high levels of glucocorticoid receptors, which makes it more vulnerable to long-term stress than most other areas of the Brain. Because the hippocampus is the most common part of the Brain where neurogenesis occurs from exercise, it has received much of the attention from scientists.

Humans are not the only animals in which exercise causes neurogenesis. Indeed, much research has been done on other animals, most commonly mice, in which scientists can use more invasive methods to determine what's going on inside the Brain in response to exercise. (The current evidence for neurogenesis in humans is indirect, using imaging techniques, since it can only be directly assessed in postmortem tissue.)

There is a strong relationship between both aerobic and resistance exercise and neurogenesis in mice.[54-57] Mice given access to a running wheel have more than twice the number of new cells formed in their Brains compared to mice with no access to a running wheel. One study even found that neurogenesis occurs, albeit to a lesser degree, when a running wheel was in the mouse cage but was locked so that the mice were not able to run on it. That the mice were still able to grab and play on the running wheel led the scientists to suggest that the wheel is stimulating enough to cause neurogenesis, although running on it caused more. Other research on mice has also shown that more running causes more neurogenesis. In a study that compared exercise-induced neurogenesis in the hippocampus of twelve different genetically divergent mouse strains, the distance run per day was significantly correlated with the density of new neurons in all mice, however, the mice that ran more had a significantly greater increase in neurogenesis compared to the mice that ran less.[58] In the mouse strain that ran the least, running increased neurogenesis by 1.6-fold, while most strains exhibited at least a doubling of neurogenesis, and the mouse strains that ran the most exhibited a four- to five-fold increase. Interestingly, physical activity was not correlated with neurogenesis in the mice housed in cages without running wheels, which suggests that exercise must reach a certain threshold level before it can have a measurable impact on neurogenesis, likely a level that stresses aerobic capacity enough to have a meaningful impact on fitness.

Having a lot of neurons is great, but it's not enough. Those neurons need to talk to one another. The way they do so is via a synapse, a physical connection linking neuron to neuron (or to a target cell) that permits a neuron to pass an electrical or chemical signal to another neuron (or to a target cell, like a muscle cell).

Synapses are important in the formation of memory. As neurotransmitters (chemical messengers that transmit a message from one nerve cell to another across the synapse) activate receptors on the target neuron that is being spoken to, the connection between the two neurons is strengthened when both neurons are active. The strength of two connected neural pathways results in the storage of information, resulting in memory.

While the hippocampus is the most common region of the Brain in which neurogenesis occurs in response to exercise, other regions are also positively affected by exercise through increases in synaptic and structural proteins, including those regions that are involved in motor control and are commonly affected by injuries and neurodegenerative disorders—the cerebellum, substantia nigra, striatum, motor cortex, and reticular formation.[59]

Like neurogenesis is to neurons, synaptogenesis is to synapses: the formation of new synapses between neurons. With more neurons and more synapses between them, the better and quicker the communication inside your Brain. And like neurogenesis, exercise causes synaptogenesis by inducing changes in a number of genes that regulate synapses, which increases synaptic connections and synaptic and structural proteins. Both neurogenesis and synaptogenesis from exercise improve memory.

As with the loss of neurons, the loss of synapses is the sign of an aging or damaged Brain. Decreases in synaptic proteins correlate with the cognitive decline observed in the Brains of individuals with Alzheimer's disease. But as with the case of neurons, exercise can "save" your synapses and improve Brain health.

"Animal models have shown that exercise reduces the extent of damage after Brain injury," says Carl Cotman, PhD, neuroscientist and founding director of the Institute for Brain Aging and Dementia at the University of California–Irvine. "Furthermore, human studies suggest that exercise can delay the onset of Alzheimer's disease. No other behavioral or pharmaceutical intervention can make such claims. Although some may exert neuroprotective or neuroplasticity effects, no other intervention has yet been shown to successfully influence both of these endpoints."

Christiane Wrann, PhD, is an assistant professor of medicine at the Cardiovascular Research Center at Massachusetts General Hospital and in the Department of Cell Biology at Harvard Medical School. Her research focuses on the molecular mechanisms behind the effects of exercise on the Brain to identify novel therapeutic targets to combat cognitive impairment in aging and neurodegenerative diseases. To dissect the effects of exercise on different aspects of Brain function—neurogenesis, synaptic plasticity, learning, and memory—Wrann and her colleagues use a variety of genetic mouse models and cutting-edge technologies, including RNA sequencing, high-resolution mass spectrometry, and advanced molecular-based screenings.

In one of Wrann's studies, in which mice ran on a running wheel daily as much as they wanted for thirty days, she discovered that several genes were activated in the hippocampus of their Brains that promote many aspects of Brain development.[60] One of these genes, brain-derived neurotrophic factor (BDNF), which encodes the protein of the same name, acts on specific neurons of the central and peripheral nervous systems, supporting the survival of existing neurons and encouraging growth and differentiation of new neurons and synapses. BDNF is synthesized in the cell body of neurons and moves back and forth to synapses, where communication between neurons occurs. BDNF is vital to learning and long-term memory and is one of the main factors responsible for exercise-induced neuroplasticity. An increase in BDNF after both acute and chronic exercise is a robust finding among research studies and is considered the main factor mediating the effects of exercise on neurogenesis, cognition, and mood.[61,62]

Another gene that Wrann discovered was upregulated in the wheel-running mice is PGC-1α, which is responsible for the formation and maintenance of specific parts of dendrites (called *spines*) in the neurons of the hippocampus. The dendrites' spines receive input from an axon at the synapse and help transmit the electrochemical stimulation received from other neurons to the cell body of the neuron to which the dendrites' spines are attached.

In addition to observing an increased activation of BDNF and PGC-1α in the hippocampus from exercise, Wrann discovered that the activation of these genes in the Brain is quantitatively comparable to their activation in skeletal muscle from exercise. In other words, exercise activates these genes in both Body (muscle) and Brain to similar degrees. And, as they do in the Brain, both BDNF and PGC-1α play prominent roles in the Body. For example, BDNF influences multiple cells involved in carbohydrate metabolism and metabolic energy balance, including pancreatic cells, liver cells, and skeletal muscle cells, all of which ultimately affect the amount of glucose in your blood.[63] And the activation of PGC-1α from exercise causes the synthesis of mitochondria (the part of the muscle responsible for aerobic metabolism), which improves the aerobic endurance of skeletal muscles.

When I first moved to southern California, I was amazed at the number of highways. The great thing about many highways is that you never need to drive very far on local roads to get to your destination. You get off the highway at one of its many exits and you're close to where you need to go. If you had to drive on local roads all the time, it would take much longer to get anywhere.

Capillaries, the smallest of blood vessels, are your muscles' and other organs' highway system. They surround and traverse your muscle fibers and organs like spider webs. Oxygen molecules in the blood "drive" along the capillaries, waiting to take an exit.

With few capillaries perfusing your muscles and other organs, oxygen molecules must travel a far distance from an exit to get to their destination—the mitochondria, the microscopic energy factories where aerobic metabolism takes place. But if there are many capillaries, oxygen molecules don't need to travel very far to get to the mitochondria. The larger the highway system of capillaries surrounding your muscles and other organs, the shorter the distance oxygen must travel from the capillaries to the mitochondria and the greater the total blood vessel surface area for oxygen diffusion.

One of the more elegant adaptations to aerobic exercise is a growth of capillaries that surround your muscle fibers, called *angiogenesis*. Indeed, aerobic exercise is one of the few physiological circumstances that cause angiogenesis, with just a few weeks of exercise needed to significantly increase the capillary content of your muscles.

Angiogenesis is a complex process requiring a lot of microscopic construction. To learn a little about that process, we need to go to England. Stuart Egginton, PhD, is the chair of exercise science in the School of Biomedical Sciences at the University of Leeds. His laboratory, along with the Angiogenesis Research Group at the University of Birmingham, where Egginton was before Leeds, studies the mechanisms underlying blood vessel growth in skeletal and cardiac muscle, including the mechanical factors associated with the physical environment of endothelial cells.

Egginton's research has provided the majority of evidence for elucidating the physiological factors of angiogenesis. Angiogenesis occurs from shear stress to the endothelial cells that line the walls of capillaries from the constant "push" of blood through them, mechanical stress to capillaries from muscle contraction, and increased muscle metabolism. Single capillaries split into two and new vessels sprout from existing capillaries, creating a larger highway system for delivering oxygen to the muscles.[64] "Angiogenesis is a complex, multifactorial process that is regulated in different ways among vascular beds and, according to the stimulus, often involving proliferation and migration of endothelial cells to form new capillaries from pre-existing vessels," Egginton says.

That complex process begins with the activation of the growth factor protein called vascular endothelial growth factor (VEGF), which is stored in vesicles in skeletal muscle cells. Research has shown that VEGF secretion from skeletal muscle is an essential step in the process of capillary growth.[65–67] Angiogenesis ultimately increases the blood vessel surface area around your muscle fibers to optimize gas exchange between your muscles and your blood—oxygen travels from your blood to your muscles and carbon dioxide and other metabolites travel from your muscles to your blood to be transported to other places.

Angiogenesis is not just specific to the vessels around your muscle fibers when you run around your neighborhood; it also occurs in your Brain.[68] Increasing blood flow to your Brain improves oxygen delivery to your Brain, just as it does in your muscles, and is one of the key mechanisms that scientists believe enhance neuroplasticity, improving cognitive functions like learning and memory, and reducing the risk of dementia as you age.[69–71]

As it does with BDNF, exercise increases VEGF. From peripheral cells, VEGF readily passes through the blood-brain barrier, causing angiogenesis in your Brain, as it does in your muscles, and interacts with BDNF to cause neurogenesis. Angiogenesis and neurogenesis are thus coupled—the two measures of Brain plasticity occur together, although angiogenesis seems to occur more quickly in response to exercise compared to neurogenesis. In some sophisticated research at the Taub Institute for Research on Alzheimer's Disease and the Aging Brain at Columbia University in New York, scientists compared MRI measurements of cerebral blood volume in mice and humans as a result of exercise-induced angiogenesis to postmortem measurements of neurogenesis in mice, and found that the increased cerebral blood volume was able to predict the amount of neurogenesis, thereby linking indirect imaging with direct, postmortem measurements.[72]

—◆—

You can't be a runner without hearing of the infamous runner's high. Even people who don't exercise have heard of it; it has become part of the English-speaking vernacular. For a long time, the source of the runner's high was (and still is among the public) linked to endorphins, with their morphine-like attributes.[73] While the level of endorphins increases in blood plasma two- to five-fold after aerobic exercise, they can barely enter the Brain through the blood-brain barrier, so it is difficult to assess whether endorphins are the reason why runners are in a happy mood after they run.

Research using radioactive tracers and positron emission tomography (PET) scans has shown that sustained moderate- and high-intensity aerobic exercise—running being the most-often studied—activates opioid and cannabinoid receptors, releasing these chemicals in the frontolimbic region of the Brain. There is a strong correlation between opioids and cannabinoids in the Brain and the perceived euphoria experienced by runners.[74,75]

Opioids and cannabinoids are psychologically rewarding and can cause reduced anxiety and a general feeling of well-being. They also buffer pain while enduring high levels of discomfort, which fosters mental toughness and self-efficacy, the belief that you can accomplish what you set out to accomplish. The opioid/cannabinoid activation—the runner's high—is one of the ways in which exercise makes you feel good about yourself, gives you confidence, and makes you mentally tough.

Evolution's natural selection may have used opioids and cannabinoids to reward large amounts of voluntary exercise, especially running.[76] Like addictive drugs, running causes neurochemical and structural adaptations in the Brain's reward pathways. The fact that exercise provides a psychological high encourages you to "just do it," and just doing it makes your Body fitter and more resilient and able to withstand environmental stressors, whether being chased by a wild animal or giving a public speech. Thus, natural selection may have provided a cool trick that encourages humans to be physically active. (On a side note, this may be the same reason why sex feels so good—to strongly encourage you to do it. The orgasm, or at least the anticipation of it, is evolution's way of ensuring reproductive success of the species.)

Through the several mechanisms by which exercise exerts its influence on your Brain—neurogenesis, synaptogenesis, angiogenesis, and genes and proteins like BDNF, PGC-1α, and VEGF—it improves Brain health; counteracts Brain disorders; improves intelligence, memory, and creativity; and prevents cognitive decline in old age.

With all this talk about how training the Body changes the Brain and improves cognition, what does that say about individuals who cannot move their bodies? Perhaps the strongest evidence for the connection between the Body and the Brain and the importance of physical movement to think and learn comes from research on individuals with spinal cord injury. A dramatic and significant change takes place in individuals' cognition as well as the perception of their lives, from before to after their injury.[77]

Many studies have reported cognitive decline in individuals after spinal cord injury. Indeed, the risk of an adult with spinal cord injury having cognitive impairment is nearly thirteen times that of someone without spinal cord injury.[78] That was the disheartening conclusion of Ashley Craig, PhD, a professor of rehabilitation studies at the University of Sydney in New South Wales, Australia, when he and his colleagues assessed cognition in 150 people with chronic spinal cord injury and compared them to able-bodied people. Craig, whose long history of research focuses on cognition and psychology following neurological injury, such as spinal cord injury and traumatic Brain injury, assessed cognitive function across five domains, including attention, memory, executive, visuoconstructional (the coordination of fine motor skills with spatial abilities), and language. In each of these cognitive domains, individuals with spinal cord injury had poorer cognitive capacity than able-bodied individuals, even when controlling for age, sex, and years of education.

In another study by the Traumatic Brain Injury Research wing of the Kessler Foundation in West Orange, New Jersey, scientists compared several areas of cognition among sixty individuals with spinal cord injury to thirty individuals of the same age (30 to 40 years old) without spinal cord injury and to twenty older individuals (50 to 60 years old) without spinal cord injury.[79] The spinal-cord injury individuals showed cognitive deficits in information processing speed, new learning, and verbal fluency compared to the age-matched healthy individuals, but exhibited similar cognition to the older healthy individuals. Other indices of cognition, including attention, working memory, and memory retrieval were not affected in the spinal-cord injury individuals.

Reviewing all studies on the subject, scientists at the University of British Columbia in Vancouver, Canada, found that in twenty-one studies that made cognitive comparisons of spinal-cord injured individuals with able-bodied individuals, fifteen showed impaired cognition.[80] In forty-nine studies that did not include able-bodied individuals, twenty-three showed significant impairments in cognitive function compared to normal population data.

Individuals who have lost their ability to move their bodies don't only experience cognitive decline; they also experience psychological changes. Craig's research and that of others has shown that many such individuals suffer from mental health problems, including depression, anxiety, stress, and post-traumatic stress disorder, especially after being discharged from inpatient rehabilitation and returning to living in the community.[81,82] While it may seem obvious and even predictable that having a major accident that causes immobility or paralysis (or even experiencing immobility from something other than a single traumatic accident) can result in depression and anxiety, it nonetheless boldly underscores the solely physical nature of human life. When we lose the ability to move the Body, we lose our Chief Executive Officer, and mental health—the functioning of the Brain and the Mind—rapidly declines.

Jon stared at me with his hazel eyes, the color nearly matching that of the sunset reflection on the silver skyscrapers outside his office window. I could tell that he was listening intently.

"It sounds like the balance between the Body and the Brain is the secret to success," Jon said.

"To live life fully, Jon," I said, "you need to see the Body and the Brain being interconnected parts of the same entity, of the same human experience. When you do, you can know all that needs to be known.

"The Body and the Brain are two parts of the same physical living being. Just because there is something unique about human cognition doesn't mean that the Brain is independent from the Body. Our efforts to understand the nature of the human Brain should, therefore, be commensurate with our efforts to understand the nature of the Body and, ultimately, the nature of life.

"Your heart, your muscles, your Brain, and all your other organs are all parts. They mean little by themselves. You can't understand the value of life's process by separating the parts from the process, or the process from the parts. When you separate the parts from the process, there is no process; there are only parts. Parts without a process have no motion, no purpose. They're lifeless. Instead of being like life, filled with motion and purpose, they are the antithesis of life.

"To fully understand the role each part plays in your life, Jon, in the way you see and interact with the world, you have to see the

Brain as part of your whole physical existence, not separate from the whole, not working at your desk by itself. Your Brain never works by itself, Jon. Never."

I paused to see how Jon would react. He started to reach for the Coca-Cola can on his desk, but stopped, pulling his arm back.

"People tend to think that the Brain sits atop the pyramid, controlling the Body, but it's actually the other way around. The Body is the Chief Executive Officer, and the Brain is the Chief Operating Officer.

"While the Brain oversees your Body's entire operation, it works in service to your Body. That's what it evolved to do. Your Brain evolved from your Body's movements to regulate your Body and manage its physiology so that it can efficiently move and interact with the world around you. Walking and running on two legs, which evolved from the anatomical change in the pelvis and is among the most complex and sophisticated of all physical movements, was the basis for the evolution of your Brain. Physical activity is so essential to your Brain that it is imperative for it to function properly.

"While the cells in your other organs, like your heart and kidneys, perform their assigned functions and don't represent any other cells or functions, the cells of your Brain represent and even control functions occurring elsewhere in your Body. The Brain works with your heart, with your kidneys, with your muscles, with your lungs, with your blood vessels, with your sensory neurons on your fingertips, and with every other part of your Body to create your physical existence, to enable the whole process to work.

"And it works the process by converting inputs from all its neurons, synapses, and neurotransmitters to outputs to create the thoughts, ideas, and perceptions that make up your Mind."

Chapter Three

Mind

IF I HAD NOT BEEN GIVEN THE GIFT OF SOMETHING SO ORDINARY, MY LIFE WOULD HAVE EVOLVED IN A COMPLETELY DIFFERENT AND MUCH MORE MUNDANE MANNER

As you walk into the Human Performance Laboratory on the campus of the University of Calgary, nestled in the shadows of the Canadian Rockies, the first thing you see is five lanes of running space that span the length of the room. Force platforms are built into the rubberized floor, and cameras on tripods surround the area. People run on the track, first with running shoes, then in bare feet—the force platforms measuring how much force is applied at different parts of the foot under these conditions—and the cameras capture every angle of the runner's movements to create a three-dimensional picture that will be analyzed using motion-analysis software.

In another room, an athlete runs on a treadmill while breathing through a snorkel-like mouthpiece, which is connected to a hose that is connected to metabolic gas analyzers that measure the volume of oxygen the athlete consumes and the amount of carbon dioxide he exhales. Every 3 minutes, a research assistant draws blood from a catheter in a vein in the athlete's arm to measure the concentration of specific metabolites, including glucose, hydrogen ions, and lactate.

In a different part of the laboratory, the research quickly changes from whole-Body movement to microscopic muscle. Walter Herzog, PhD, an imposingly tall, thin man and director of the Human Performance Laboratory, stands among some sophisticated equipment.

"We're identifying the molecular mechanisms of muscle contraction," Herzog says in his Swiss German accent, as if it's just another day at the office.

Herzog is one of the world's top scientists in the fascinating and wide-reaching field of biomechanics, which merges the physics and biology of human movement. His faculty position at the University of Calgary traverses a few departments, including kinesiology, mechanical engineering, and medicine. His main emphasis of research these days is on the neuro-biomechanics of skeletal muscle. His laboratory was the first and is only one of two laboratories in the world to isolate and mechanically test properties of isolated sarcomeres, the repeated sections that run the length of muscle proteins, which are the smallest units of muscle contraction. His research is shedding new light on how the proteins inside muscles work together to cause muscle contraction.

In 2006, Herzog won the prestigious Borelli Award, which, fittingly, is named after the seventeenth century scientist Giovanni Alphonso Borelli, whose book, *De Motu Animalium* (*Of Animal Motion*), is perhaps the oldest documentation of a scientific study of running. It's fitting because Herzog is not just a great scholar. He's also a lifelong runner. His favorite race is 800 meters, the metric equivalent of a half-mile.

"Running twice around the track as fast as I can has fascinated me for many years," he says.

At 67 years old, Herzog has been running ever since he can remember. He grew up speaking German in Bad Zurzach, a town of two-and-a-half square miles on the Rhein River in the northern part of Switzerland. His first race was at the age of 6, when he competed in a 60-meter sprint race. He was the fastest kid in town, although he jokes that the town had only sixteen boys his age, so it wasn't that hard to be the fastest. But running for Herzog wasn't just about being fast.

"From very early on as a kid, I realized that my bodily and spiritual well-being—my Body and my Brain—were one and the same and intricately connected."

Like for many kids growing up in Switzerland, most of the running Herzog did was while playing soccer. He played competitive soccer from the age of 7 and then entered local races—sprints, cross-country, and on the road.

"The first time I realized that I probably had a bit of talent for running was when I went to the Swiss Age-Group Championships at age 12, and I won the 600-meter race and placed second in the high jump and long jump without any formal training, only with soccer games that lasted all Saturday afternoon," he says. "I probably ran 10 to 20 kilometers [6 to 12 miles] during those games."

At age 14, still playing soccer but without any formal run training, he competed again at the Swiss Age-Group Championships and placed fifth, breaking 3 minutes in the 1,000-meter run, and placed third in both the shot put and long jump. At 17, he joined an official track club for the first time and ran 800 meters in 2:04. At 18, he ran 1:57, and at 19, he ran 1:52. Later that year, he and his two best friends won the 3 × 1,000-meter relay at the Swiss National Championships, setting the Swiss record that stood for many years.

When Herzog turned 20, his goal was to run 800 meters in 1:48, which was about 4 seconds off the world record at that time. Having run "only" 1:51, he decided to study full-time and forget about his international and Olympic ambitions. "I felt that I was a couple of seconds too slow to ever be competitive on the international level," he says.

He continued training three to five times per week, going on half-hour runs and a couple of track workouts each week in the summer, and continued to run 800 meters between 1:51 and 1:53 on moderate training until he was 28 years old. Then, he stopped running competitively. He cross-country skied throughout the winters and ran recreationally in the summers, but it would be twenty years until he would compete again on the track.

I first met Herzog when he was 40 years old. I was a 22-year-old inexperienced but overconfident master's degree student when I stepped into his office at the University of Calgary. I was both impressed and intimidated. I could tell he meant business. He revealed in a later conversation that he did not feel the same way about me and, in so many words, told me that his first impression of me was not good. It would take me the better portion of two years to change my academic advisor's opinion of me.

One day, I was sitting in Herzog's office, talking to him about the research project we were working on—the esoteric topic of muscle-fiber recruitment patterns during eccentric contractions—and I asked him how he acquired his ability to develop his own ideas about how and why muscles work the way they do.

"Years of research," he responded immediately.

It wasn't until years later, after I had experienced years of research myself while working on my own PhD, that I understood what he had meant and had reached the empowering point at which I could develop my own ideas.

After starting to compete again on the track at age 48, Herzog competed in the Masters World Track and Field Championships in Edmonton, Alberta, at age 50 "just because it was close by," he says. He placed third in the 400 meters and second in the 800 meters, running a quick 2:09 and losing by just one-hundredth of a second. He currently holds several age-group records in Alberta in the 600 and 800 meters.

At 67, Herzog says, "Running 2:20 still feels like running 1:51 when I was young. It's the same effort, feels like the same speed, and still gives me the same satisfaction as when I was 20 years old."

I couldn't help but ask him how he sees running through the eyes of a scientist, especially one who has devoted much of his career to the mechanics of muscles.

"When I cross-country ski, I think a lot of the mechanics of it, because it is so technical that, after fifty-five years of doing it, I am still getting better technically every year. When running, I never think about the mechanics or the muscles; running is just natural locomotion."

Herzog is not just a scientist who runs fast for his age, although that alone would be interesting. Being a speedy scientist is central to who Herzog is, because he wouldn't be a scientist at all if he didn't run fast.

"Having been given a bit of talent for running, it gave me the confidence for a life that I would never have found in my farming and working-class family," he says. "It opened doors and avenues that I would never have dared to explore otherwise. The fact is, if I had not been given the gift of something so ordinary, my life would have evolved in a completely different and much more mundane manner, because I would never have believed that a little kid from a little town could ever aspire to more than an ordinary working life in a small village. Running gave me confidence that I could not find anywhere else in my life. Without it, I would never have studied at university, and I would never have become an academic and a scientist. I would have become a laborer like my father, married to a local girl and happy with a little family."

Training the Body gives us something so meaningful, something so profound, that it gives a 6-year-old kid in a tiny farming village in Switzerland the confidence to leave his home country to earn a PhD and become one of the top scientists in his field in the world.

For her PhD thesis in sport psychology at Sheffield Hallam University in Sheffield, England, Kate Hays, PhD, interviewed fourteen male and female athletes from different sports who had won a medal at either the Olympic Games, World Champion-ships, or World Cup, and asked them to state where they thought their confidence in themselves as an athlete came from, to give some specific examples of the types of things they were confident about, and to describe the time that they felt most confident going into an important competition.[1] All fourteen athletes highlighted the importance of good physical preparation in making them confident. As one Olympic gold medalist in her study said, "For me, there was no doubt at all that when I felt confident, it was because I was physically in very good condition." Other studies on Olympic-level athletes have also found that physical preparation is a major factor influencing athletes' confidence and performance at the Olympics.[2]

Olympic athletes are not the only people whose confidence grows from training their Body. Many scientific studies have shown that people of all ages who exercise have greater self-esteem and self-efficacy.[3] For most people, self-confidence, and consequently their approach to life, is intimately connected to their physical being. The confidence you get from working out can pervade every other area of your life. What you think about your-self and your capabilities is arguably the most important factor in determining what actions and directions you take in your life. And it often determines how successful you are.

Even the expectation that exercise is good for your Mind is enough to make it so. In an interesting study at Université Laval in Québec, Canada, forty-four healthy, young adults par-ticipated in a supervised ten-week exercise program consisting of 90 minutes of aerobic exercise three times per week.[4] Half the participants were told that the exercise program was specifically designed to improve their psychological well-being. The participants were reminded of this throughout the program and encouraged to attend to signs of psychological improvement. For the other half of participants, the biological (fitness) aspects of the exercise program were emphasized, with no mention of any psychological benefits.

Following the ten-week program, both groups of participants had similar increases in aerobic fitness. However, the participants who were told that the exercise was designed to increase psychological well-being perceived their exercise program as more psychologically effective, showed a significant improvement in self-esteem, and exhibited a greater increase in self-esteem compared to the other group.

What research like this suggests is that simply by reading a book on how creating a sound Body creates a sound Mind, it can do just that, as long as you believe it. While the Body wants to move and the Brain wants to supervise, the Mind is responsible for your thoughts and beliefs.

But you still have to act on those beliefs.

While there are plenty of mindfulness gurus and books claiming that success starts with a belief, success does not and cannot start that way. As Herzog's and others' lives have shown, success starts with the physical act. Seeing results from the physical act is what *makes* us believe. We don't believe gravity exists and then see an object drop to the ground from our hand when we let go of it. We see an object drop to the ground from our hand when we let go of it and then we believe gravity exists. And so it is with many other phenomena: We believe what we *see*.

As a lifelong runner and coach, I see this all the time. What gives runners confidence, what makes them believe they can reach their goals, is their physical achievements. A belief without evidence to support that belief is simply blind faith. For good runners, the physical achievement may be running a specific type of workout faster than what had been done before. When workouts go well, runners' heads are filled with positivity, and they believe they will run a faster race. And then they do. Conversely, when workouts don't go well, runners lose confidence. They get down on themselves, start to think they're not fit, and their heads are filled with negativity. In those moments, there's little I can say as a coach to negate or detract from their observation of a subpar physical performance to make them believe differently. Because they believe what they *see*.

For beginner runners, the physical achievement may be being able to run 1 mile. Many beginner runners have trouble believing that running a marathon is possible. It seems daunting at first. But then they sign up for a marathon program and start training. As the weeks and months pass, they run 5 miles, 10 miles, 15 miles, 20 miles. With each milestone, the belief that running a marathon is possible becomes stronger.

You don't need to be a runner to believe and be affected by what you see. Many (most?) people believe things about themselves based on their perceptions of their Bodies, especially their Body weight. The extreme case of this is Body dysmorphia, a mental health disorder that makes people obsess over what they perceive as defects or flaws in their Bodies. Body dysmorphia can affect every part of a person's life.

It's always the physical that comes first. We believe what we see.

Because the Body controls the Mind and therefore the physical act comes first—just like it did for our ancient ancestors—you don't need to believe that you'll be successful at something before acting at or on that something. You need only to act first. As Richard Pascale, Jerry Sternin, and Monique Sternin wrote in *The Power of Positive Deviance*, "It's easier to act your way into a new way of thinking than to think your way into a new way of acting."

Not everyone has thought that the Body controls the Mind, or even that they are connected. Philosophers and scholars as far back as the ancient Greeks described humans as being composed of two distinct parts: Mind and Body. Plato believed that the

Mind is the only true reality, the thing of greatest worth, that ideas are implanted in the Mind before they are embedded in the Body. All these years later, many people still see the Body and the Mind as distinct parts of the whole human being. As philosopher Mark Johnson, PhD, of the University of Oregon wrote in *The Meaning of the Body: Aesthetics of Human Understanding*:[5]

> *Although most people never think about it very carefully, they live their lives assuming and acting according to a set of dichotomies that distinguish mind from body, reason from emotion, and thought from feeling. Mind/body dualism is so deeply embedded in our philosophical and religious traditions, in our shared conceptual systems, and in our language that it can seem to be an inescapable fact about human nature.*

Far be it for me to argue with Plato, perhaps the most famous philosopher ever, but the Body and the Mind are not two distinct parts of the human being; they are intimately connected.

How they are connected is a bit of a problem, one that other famous philosophers have been trying to solve for centuries. The Mind, as French philosopher René Descartes claimed, is not physically connected to the Body because the Mind is not a physical object like the Body and therefore cannot and does not take up space. However, the Body, like all matter, is spatial. It takes up space, with characteristics such as height, length, and depth. Where the real problem lies is not in the *difference* between the Body and the Mind, but in the *way* in which they are different—the Body taking up space and the Mind not—which makes their interaction impossible because, for the two to interact, what is in space must act on what is not in space and vice versa. For example, if your Mind decides on spaghetti and meatballs for dinner, spaghetti and meatballs don't automatically present themselves on your dinner plate.

How can something that is not physical interact with and act on something that is?

The Brain.

Remember that the Brain is the Chief Operating Officer of your existence. It directs and manages the entire operation, taking its cue from the Body, the Chief Executive Officer.

Training the Body changes the Brain, which affects the Mind.

But even the Brain—acting as the physical connection between the Body and the Mind—doesn't completely solve the Mind-Body problem. After all, how can all the insightful thoughts, creative imaginations, and empathic emotions that make up the human Mind arise from the Brain's mushy gray matter and the connections between its neurons?

Your Mind is made up of your thoughts, emotions, perceptions, and language, all of which are parts of your biological chemistry. As such, the Mind does, indeed, exist in the Body—your living organism—and not as an abstract phenomenon, separate from the Body, as Plato and Descartes claimed. The difference between Body and Mind is one of degree and not of kind. While Descartes's famous mantra, *"Cogito, ergo sum"*—"I think, therefore I am"—suggests that thinking about one's existence is proof in itself that one exists to do the thinking (as Descartes himself explained, "We cannot doubt of our existence while we doubt"), it is your physical matter—the Brain—that determines what your Mind is and what it can become. Many other animals have a Mind and the ability to form thoughts. However, because they don't possess sophisticated language, they lack the ability to communicate their thoughts to others and to themselves.

As an athlete growing up in rural Switzerland, Walter Herzog is not the first person or even the first scientist to recognize the Mind-Body connection. Hippocrates, commonly considered the Father of Medicine, wrote in *On the Sacred Disease* in 400 BC:[6]

Men ought to know that from the brain, and from the brain only, arise our pleasures, joy, laughter and jests, as well as our sorrows, pains, grief and tears. Through it, in particular,

we think, see, hear, and distinguish the ugly from the beauti-
ful, the bad from the good, the pleasant from the unpleasant
. . . wherefore I assert that the brain is the interpreter of
consciousness.

Like Hippocrates, Aristotle also believed the Body and the Mind are intertwined. There can be no matter without Mind, he proposed, and no Mind without matter. The Mind itself exists within matter—the Brain, which is the vessel that contains the electrical impulses that create the Mind.

And training the Body with physical activity stimulates and changes the Brain's electrical impulses, which affects the Mind. As Roman philosopher Marcus Cicero claimed in 65 BC, "'tis exercise alone that supports the spirits, and keeps the mind in vigor."[7] In the 1800s, American philosopher Henry David Thoreau said of walking, "The moment my legs begin to move my thoughts begin to flow, as if I had given vent to the stream at the lower end and consequently new fountains flowed into it at the upper."[8]

Since the Body is involved in everything you do, it is critically important for what and how you think. Scientists call this *embodied cognition*. The research of developmental and social psychologists has shown that the Body, along with its environment, plays a central role in your perceptions and in the development of intelligence.[9] Indeed, the Body is a grounding mechanism for how we think about abstract concepts. For example, when you think about a past event in your life, like your first kiss or the first time you drove a car, your Body is likely to sway backward; when you think about a future event, like your birthday party or a vacation, your Body is likely to sway forward.[10] Even though past and future events have nothing to do with physical space, your Body naturally associates them with a physical attribute, by swaying backward (to embody the past) and forward (to embody the future).

Manipulating parts of your Body, including your face, head, arms, and torso, not only affects your thinking abilities, such as evaluation, decision-making, and attribution, it *causes* you to think (and subsequently act) in a particular way.[11,12] Bodily behaviors, such as making a fist with your hand or sitting with a certain posture, affect how others perceive you and how you perceive yourself.[13] These perceptions are then translated into specific behaviors. For example, if you sit in a chair with an expanded posture while talking to someone, the other person is likely to perceive you as being dominant and will assume a constricted posture, as if to be submissive (and vice versa), without being aware of his or her perception or corresponding behavior.[14]

Think about when you nod your head as if to say "yes" when having a conversation with someone. You're more likely to have a positive attitude toward what that person is saying than if you were to shake your head as if you were saying "no." And if you held a heavy weight in your hand, you would be more likely to judge or value something as more important compared to when holding a light weight. This latter quirky characteristic was the interesting finding of scientists at the University of Amsterdam, who had people hold heavy and light clipboards and asked them several types of questions related to cognition—estimation of the value of foreign currencies, the importance of having a voice in making decisions, value judgments about their city and its mayor, and evaluation of weak and strong arguments about a particular issue.[15] In all four conditions, people's thoughts were influenced by the heaviness of the clipboard, such that people placed more value and importance on things when holding the heavier weight compared to the lighter weight. The scientists concluded that "much as weight makes people invest more physical effort in dealing with concrete objects, it also makes people invest more cognitive effort in dealing with abstract issues."

Changes in perception are not limited to how much weight you hold in your hand. If you're standing at the bottom of a hill and are asked how steep it is, your answer will depend on how physically fit you are. Such was the conclusion of researchers at the University of Virginia, who asked seventy-four athletes and nonathletes to judge the steepness of four hills of 5, 6, 21, and 31 degrees.[16] The less physically fit the individual, the steeper he or she perceived the hills to be compared to their actual steepness. In addition to physical fitness, several other Body-centered factors influenced visual perception of hill steepness. As the scientists showed in their series of studies on the topic, hills look steeper to people wearing a heavy backpack, who are physically fatigued, who are elderly, or who are in poor physical health.

Perception based on factors relating to the Body is not exclusive to the steepness of a hill; embodied perception—and the physical effort anticipated—also influences horizontal distance.[17,18] Your Body influences the way your Brain perceives the outside world, and those perceptions change as your Body changes. As the researchers stated, "Conscious slant perception is malleable and changes as the physiological potential of the observer changes, regardless of whether these changes are long or short term."[19]

Beyond how the Body affects cognition, intelligence, and perception is its effects on psychology. Psychologist Sigmund Freud believed that the Body is the core of an individual's psychological identity. As most people know when they look in the mirror, physical appearance is related to emotional well-being, happiness, and self-esteem. The human psychological experience is intimately connected to a sense of one's Body because it is impossible to separate the Body from the Brain and from the Mind. Research has shown that individuals who exercise a lot and individuals with good physical health have higher levels of psychological well-being than those who exercise less and have poor physical health.[20]

Although having a more highly developed Brain inside your skull compared to other animals enables you to dream things and imagine things and do things that other animals can't, your sophisticated Brain doesn't come without side effects. Having such sophisticated Brains makes humans vulnerable to many psychiatric conditions, with depression and anxiety being the most common. Depression affects more than 340 million people worldwide and is the world's leading cause of disability.

Examining the Brain in both living individuals and in those after death has revealed that those with depression and anxiety disorders have atrophy or loss of neurons in the hippocampus and prefrontal cortex.[21,22] Strategies to cause neurogenesis can, therefore, mitigate depression and anxiety. Neurogenesis is one of the primary ways to reduce depression and is one of the ways by which antidepressant medications work.

To test whether an increase in neurogenesis is *required* for antidepressants to work, scientists at the Center for Neurobiology and Behavior at Columbia University gave mice three types of antidepressants, an antipsychotic drug, or a placebo vehicle used as a control treatment, and assessed their feeding behavior.[23] (Antidepressants are known to affect appetite.) After five days, the mice treated with antidepressants showed no effect on latency to feed relative to the vehicle-treated mice. (A vehicle is a substance, such as saline or mineral oil, to deliver the experimental treatment, like the applesauce that your mother used as a vehicle to give you medicine when you were a kid.) After twenty-eight days, however, all three antidepressants (but not the antipsychotic drug) caused significant decreases in latency to feed.

To test if hippocampal neurogenesis participates in the mechanism by which antidepressants act, the scientists then disrupted the process by giving the mice radiation to the hippocampus to kill its neurons, treated the mice with antidepressants or vehicle control, and again assessed their feeding behavior. Surprisingly, the scientists found that disrupting antidepressant treatment caused a significant reduction in latency to feed in the vehicle-treated mice, but not in mice treated with radiation, and radiation did not affect latency to feed in the vehicle-treated mice. Antidepressant-induced neurogenesis is a *requirement* to mitigate depression and blocks the behavioral responses to antidepressants.[24]

Neurogenesis not only helps you to think more creatively or improve your intelligence; it is the trick to mitigating depression.

It has been known since the 1980s in the scientific and medical communities that aerobic exercise is just as, if not more, effective as prescription antidepressants in mitigating depression.[25] The two main ways by which exercise does so are stimulating neurogenesis and increasing serotonin in the Brain.[26] In addition to a loss of neurons, clinically depressed individuals have chronically low serotonin in the Brain. Serotonin is a powerful neurotransmitter (a type of chemical that relays signals from one area of the Brain to another) responsible for feelings of well-being and happiness. It directly or indirectly influences most of your Brain cells. When serotonin is low, you're more likely to get depressed.

Aerobic exercise is so important in reducing depression that depression is inversely related to an individual's maximum aerobic capacity—the higher the aerobic fitness, the lower the depression.[27] The relationship also works the other way—individuals with depressive symptoms are more likely than those without depressive symptoms to have poor exercise capacity. One study on people with heart disease found that, for each standard deviation increase in depression score, the odds of having poor exercise capacity increased by 20 percent, even when other factors related to their heart disease were considered.[28]

There is yet another way in which exercise mitigates depression. Reducing Body fat.

Scientists at the University of Hong Kong discovered that the antidepressant effects of exercise are mediated partly by the exercise-induced production of adiponectin, a protein hormone secreted by fat cells that crosses the blood-brain barrier and promotes neurogenesis in the hippocampus.[29] Adiponectin, which is increased with exercise, modulates several metabolic processes, including glucose regulation in the blood and the oxidation of fat in the liver and skeletal muscle. It also possesses antidiabetic, anti-inflammatory, antiatherogenic, and cardioprotective properties. Adiponectin is inversely correlated with body-fat percentage: The lower your body-fat percentage, the higher your level of adiponectin. Thus, it appears that reducing your body-fat percentage with exercise increases adiponectin, which causes neurogenesis in your Brain.

—◆—

If you have ever run with someone who is much fitter than you, you've seen how easy the run is for that person, while you're huffing and puffing, feeling like your heart is pounding out of your chest. When a physically fit person and unfit person exercise at the same intensity, the unfit person experiences significantly more stress than does the fit person. The higher your level of physical fitness, the greater your ability to tolerate high workloads and be minimally stressed by low ones. This is also true when dealing with the stresses of life: When you're unfit, even a small life stress can have big consequences, on both your Mind and your health. To find out why, we need to visit Chicago, Germany, and Bethesda, Maryland.

At the Human Behavioral Pharmacology Laboratory at the University of Chicago, there is a research laboratory that looks like a living room. In the room is an easy chair for relaxing, a television and video player, and a desk with a computer. It is where Emma Childs, PhD, an associate professor of psychiatry, conducts her research.

In one of her studies, 111 individuals participated in two experimental sessions in that room at least 48 hours apart in randomized order: one with a stressful task and one with a non-stressful task that served as the control condition.[30] The stressful task consisted of a 5-minute speech and 5 minutes of mental arithmetic, which was video recorded in front of two research assistants who were strangers to the participants and provided no feedback. The video of the participants was projected onto a television screen during the task. For the non-stressful control task, the participants spoke to the research assistant for 5 minutes about a favorite book, movie, or TV show, then played Solitaire on the computer for 5 minutes, with no video camera recording them.

Childs and her colleagues measured the participants' heart rate, blood pressure, the stress hormone cortisol, and mood before and several times after the two tasks. They also documented the amount of exercise the participants normally did to compare measures between those who exercised and those who didn't.

As expected, Childs found that the stressful task significantly increased heart rate, blood pressure, and cortisol among all participants compared to the non-stressful control task. The stressful task also significantly increased negative mood characteristics (anxiety, depression, anger, and confusion) and decreased positive mood characteristics (friendliness, elation, and positivity). However, individuals who exercised regularly exhibited less of a decline in positive mood characteristics from the stressful task than did the non-exercising individuals, and the non-exercising individuals had significantly greater decreases in positive mood characteristics from the stress. These results led Childs to conclude that people who exercise are more resistant to acute stress.

An ability to maintain a more positive mood during stressful situations may serve a protective function, Childs says, minimizing the accumulation of stress with repeated exposures that is linked to the development of disease. Other studies have also found that exercise causes a reduced reaction to psychological stress.[31,32] It seems that habitual physical activity is associated with stress resilience.

Of course, there may be other lifestyle or cognitive factors related to a habit of exercise that could mitigate stress. To test if exercise itself reduces stress, Sandra Klaperski, PhD, and her colleagues at the University of Freiburg's Institute of Sports Science in Germany randomly assigned ninety-six individuals into three training groups for twelve weeks: (1) an aerobic exercise group, which ran outdoors at 60 to 80 percent of maximum heart rate for an hour twice per week, (2) a relaxation training group, which trained with several relaxation techniques, including muscle relaxation, breathing exercises, imagery, and passive concentration of bodily perceptions, and (3) a control group, which did not receive either of the two interventions.[33]

Before and after the twelve-week interventions, the scientists measured physical fitness and compared the groups' stress responses (salivary cortisol, heart rate, and heart rate variability) to a standardized psychosocial stress test. The aerobic exercise group significantly improved fitness and reduced stress reactivity in all three stress responses. The relaxation training group reduced only cortisol reactivity, and no changes in stress responses occurred in the control group.

We don't all have the same psychological reactions to potential stressors. As Patricia Deuster, PhD, and Marni Silverman, PhD, of the Uniformed Services University of the Health Sciences in Bethesda, Maryland, have found, exercise and fitness serve as a buffer against both physical and psychosocial stressors, which protect against stress-related disorders and chronic illnesses.[34] Exercise is a stress buffer—when you make your Body fit, strong, and enduring, you also make it resilient to stress, decreasing your risk of health issues when you encounter stress in your life. A study at the University of Kansas found that fitness moderates the relationship between stress and illness. After experiencing a year's worth of life stress, unfit individuals had poorer physical health and depression compared to fit individuals. For fit individuals, their high life stress had little impact on their subsequent physical health and depression.[35]

Why does exercise buffer against stress and create such resiliency?

Exercise makes your Brain tough.[36,37]

Aerobic exercise causes adaptations in neural circuits involved in mediating the response to stress, including growth, survival, and differentiation of neurons, transmission of Brain nerve impulses by the neurotransmitters serotonin and norepinephrine, and an increase in the neuropeptide galanin in the Brain, which correlates with and confers resilience to stress.[38]

While acute exposure to a physical stress induces a transient and predictable stress response, as described by Selye's General Adaptation Syndrome, repeated, intermittent exposure to that stress, with enough time to recover in between exposures, serves as "stress training" or "toughening." When you work out consistently, your Body makes specific microadjustments to assuage the stress.

And you connect your Body, your Brain, and your Mind.

Because your Body is not the only one that adapts. Your Brain adapts. Your Mind adapts. Pushing your Body with hard workouts, with weeks and months and years of hard training, not only changes how your Brain perceives and reacts to physical stress, it affects the way you think about the stress. Both physical and mental toughness are acquired through physical training, as you become more capable of tolerating high degrees of discomfort. You become comfortable with being uncomfortable.

And the level at which you become uncomfortable rises to a whole new level.

This physiological toughening is characterized by an initial stress neurotransmitter response (which prepares your Body for "fight-or-flight" reactions), followed by a rapid recovery, along with a reduced response from your central stress response system—the hypothalamic-pituitary-adrenal (HPA) axis—which regulates many homeostatic Body systems, including metabolism, cardiovascular system, immune system, reproductive system, and central nervous system. The exercise-mediated response of the HPA axis also exists in children as young as 8 years old.[39] "This protective physiological profile appears to be associated with improved performance during challenging or stressful situations, increased tolerance to stressors, increased emotional stability, and improved immune function," says Silverman. "Having a valid measure of physical fitness, in particular aerobic fitness, may be one of the best indicators of resilience."

Another way in which physical training makes you more resilient in the face of stress is called *cognitive reappraisal*, the deliberate viewing of an emotionally evocative event from a different (positive) perspective and reinterpreting its meaning, thereby changing its emotional impact. This remarkable ability to reappraise a stressful situation occurs even when adjusting for individuals' anxious and depressive dispositions as well as for their general creative potential.[40]

Working on your Body changes your Mind about stressful situations, influencing a more positive outlook. Research has shown that the ability to reappraise a stressful situation has to do with the recruitment of specific parts of the Brain. Individuals who have a greater capacity for reappraising stressful events are more capable or more prone to recruit the lateral prefrontal cortex when the situation demands that they come up with alternative appraisals of such events.[41]

In a social world, this skill can come in handy when dealing with others. The effect of exercise on the prefrontal cortex extends beyond the individual who exercises; it also helps you deal with other people and modify your behavior toward others. For example, a study at the University of Washington in Seattle found that physical activity significantly moderates the effects of being treated without respect or dignity by a supervisor (called *interpersonal injustice*) on the loss of ability to control oneself (called *self-regulation depletion*), and reduces the influence on social undermining directed toward the supervisor.[42] In other words, physical exercise can prevent you from losing control when dealing with a difficult boss at work who treats you unfairly and from taking actions that undermine your relationship with him or her.

Cognitive reappraisal extends beyond dealing with a stressful boss at work. Cognitive reappraisal helps us find comfort in what is, oftentimes, an uncomfortable life.

The functional MRI research corroborates what we think about when we exercise. When exercise intensity is low, thoughts tend to be *dissociative*—people think about things other than the physical activity. When exercise intensity is high, thoughts tend to be *associative*—people think about what their Body is doing and the effort they're exerting. [43,44] What modulates our internal dialogue is our perceived exertion, which influences the amount of focus required and the urgency to self-monitor physical changes and sensations. As the intensity or effort increases, we become more focused on the Body and its ability to perform the task.

I learned early in my life as a runner that when running is hard, I think about the hard; when running is easy, I think about other things.

I learned early in my life as a runner that there is value in thinking about the hard.

Exploiting the physicality of the human existence with intense physical activity helps us manage discomfort, helps us mitigate life's pain and suffering. Research using fMRI has shown that running, but not walking, attenuates the post-run sensation of externally administered pain, by interfering with a key region of the Brain's pain pathway. [45]

During those physically uncomfortable moments in every race, in every challenging workout, I am faced with a dilemma: Do I back off from the discomfort to make the experience feel better, or do I push through it to achieve the result I want and learn about myself in a unique and extraordinary way? I am asked, "What am I going to do *right now*?"

Few other times in my life am I asked such a decisive question at such a decisive moment.

Sometimes, in answering that question, I find out things about myself that make me proud. I am proud of myself for managing the discomfort in a positive way, to push past something uncomfortable to find something extraordinary. Other times, I find out things about myself that are less desirable, things I would rather not admit, things I don't really want to know. It is in those revealing moments that I learn about how I handle difficult situations. For better or for worse, I get to know who I am. If I fail or disappoint myself, I can promise myself to handle those situations better next time. And so can you.

The encounter with physical discomfort is purifying. It gives you the opportunity to test the strength of your will by providing an obstacle, and you learn to what extent you are in control of yourself. How great of a gift it is that you can use your Body to strengthen your courage and your resolve so that you can deal with pain.

You can *choose* to suffer.

The suffering Body, as the ancient Roman Stoic philosopher Seneca described, becomes an aid to self-knowledge, a route to philosophical progress. And it prepares and toughens you for the stresses of life.

It had been a week since Jon and I met. We returned to his office, nineteen floors above the street level, the sounds of the Indianapolis traffic barely audible. It was still early, the orange glow of sunset dancing on the skyscrapers of downtown still several hours away.

"I haven't run for so long that I've forgotten how to deal with discomfort," Jon said. "I miss the emotional high of a hard workout, the pain of racing, the thrill of the physical effort."

"Yes, Jon! That's exactly right," I said, excited at his comments. "The Mind—the place where you sense that emotion, that pain, that thrill—can only be understood in the context of its relationship to a physical Body that interacts with the world. We evolved from other animals whose neural processing and cognitive activity were driven primarily by their perceptions and interactions with their environment. The Mind, rather than being abstract and distinct from the Body, is deeply rooted in the Body's senses, perceptions, and movements. The Body shapes and serves the Mind.

"When you run, much more is going on than simply the muscular contractions in your legs and the sweat production on your skin. Your physical movements are how you learn about the world, how you learn about yourself. They are what enable you to produce the unity of your conscious experience."

Jon tapped his desk.

"Over millions of years, Jon, evolution has created a human Mind distinguished from all other animals, a Mind that functions both rationally and emotionally, but that is always grounded by instinct. Your Mind is an exquisite and complex instrument of survival, with millions of rich thoughts formed from the physical connections between neurons."

"I never knew my Mind worked like that," Jon said apologetically.

"I'm afraid that most people don't know," I responded.

"Because of the physical connection between your Mind and your Body, you cannot change your Mind and change your life without changing your Brain first. All those new neurons and synapses and proteins and cerebral, oxygen-rich blood flow that result from working out are what enable you to think differently. They make your Brain more adaptable.

"It all comes down to neuroplasticity.

"But Jon, that doesn't mean that if you run every day or swing heavy kettlebells in the gym, you'll be able to do differential calculus or solve difficult problems, like rush-hour traffic. Plenty of individuals work out and are, for lack of a better word, unintelligent. Not every physically fit person is smart and creative. While training your Body changes your Brain, it doesn't *automatically* affect your Mind. The cognitive improvements from exercise, with all those tiny neurons talking to each other through synapses, are much more subtle than are the changes to muscle, fat, and capil-laries. Exercise alone is not the antidote to stupidity or the trick to living a confident, successful life. But it's a good start. Because your Body itself is intelligent. It is perhaps the most intelligent organism on the planet.

"Trying to change your Mind, trying to become more creative, trying to be more confident, trying to be more resilient in the face of stress without first making the changes to your Brain doesn't work. That's like trying to build a house without having and orga-nizing the right materials to build it. You need to add the right materials to your Brain. You cannot change your Brain until you train your Body.

"When you work from the outside in, rather than from the inside out, you will live a confident, successful life. You will live life as an animal. And you will become *human*, revealing all the potential inside of you."

Jon's eyes grew wide. I could see that he got it. I could see that his Mind was racing. I could see that he was excited to start working *out* again so he could progress from where he is now to where he wanted to be, to where he believed he could be.

And he was starting to realize that he was walking around with the secret all along. All he needed to do was to act on it.

PART II

THE WORKOUTS

Many years ago, as a personal trainer in a gym, I was talking to one of the gym's members as she rode a stationary bike alongside her workout buddies. While I was explaining how she and her friends could get better results from their workouts, I sensed that she wasn't listening. Perhaps she didn't care for the advice of a young, scrawny-looking runner in cotton sweatpants. A few days later, I saw her again when I was about to go for a run. Seeing me for the first time in my running shorts, she enthusiastically asked, "How can I get legs like yours?" Smiling, I joked, "So you want me for my Body rather than for my Mind?"

It's not enough to read, or listen to a scrawny-looking runner in cotton sweatpants talk about how training your Body changes your Brain, which affects your Mind. You need to act on what you learn.

It's time to create a sound Body to create a sound Mind.

It's time to work out.

None of the workouts in this book are easy. But neither is life if you live it with passion and purpose.

The workouts described on these pages make your Body enduring, strong, powerful, and agile.

To be resilient against the stresses of life.

To interact with your environment and with other people with confidence.

To improve performance by labor and exertion, like what *work out* means.

To change your Brain.

To affect your Mind.

Many of the workouts take you outside in nature. Like an animal in the wild.

And inside yourself.

———

My conversation with Jon was coming to an end. I had shared with him everything I wanted to share. I showed him all the workouts to make his Body enduring, strong, powerful, and agile. I could see that he was becoming more confident, more at peace. His Mind was slowly changing. All that was left was to tie the parts together, for him to see how each part of him—his Body, his Brain, and his Mind—is essential and how each essential part fits within the bigger picture to create the life he wanted.

"Thank you for explaining things to me, Jason, for showing me how to train my Body, and for helping me to understand how my life starts with my Body and how important it is to be physically fit like an animal," Jon said.

"It's been my pleasure, Jon. I am confident you will apply what you have learned, and train your Body to change your Brain to affect your Mind to create the life you want.

"Because, Jon, your Mind is what sets you apart. The Body, for the most part, is the same for everyone and even for every other mammal. It's anatomy. It's biology. It's biochemistry. It's genetically granted. But your Mind is different. Your Mind is distinctly you. The Mind you have is *your* Mind; no one else can ever have the same experience of the Mind, because your experiences, your external and internal sensory perceptions, and your Brain's billions of neuronal connections are never the same as anyone else's. Your Mind is not genetically granted in completed form. You can enhance it; you can *change* it. Training your Body expands your Mind, providing the forum for ideas to develop, manifest, and grow, offering a unique space of cognitive freedom.

"What you experience in your Mind doesn't just distinguish you from all other people, Jon. It distinguishes you from all other animals and even from all other living organisms.

"Unlike any other animal, humans have a unique capacity—which is central to who we are as humans—to think about our Mind and to be mindful about our thoughts. We think about ourselves as different from others and even capable of being different from our current self. We think a future for ourselves that does not yet exist. We think a life that we have never lived. We think a self we have yet to become. Our Mind drives us to become good people and to live fulfilling lives.

"The major difference between you and a monkey, Jon, is that you have an extraordinary Mind that can think and imagine and create.

"A monkey doesn't spend time thinking about who he or she is. He doesn't spend time thinking about being the best monkey he can be. He doesn't spend time thinking about whether or not he is living up to what it means to be a monkey. He doesn't manifest living in a big monkey mansion, finding a monkey wife, and becoming partner in a monkey law firm. He doesn't ask himself, 'Am I fulfilled?' The internal conflict that we all experience does not and cannot exist in any other species. Internal conflict is a uniquely human quality.

"So when you think how close to your potential you can get and you ask yourself, 'I wonder what I could be?' that is the truly human question. It's the question that is at the heart—and in the Brain and the Mind—of being human."

Jon nodded. He didn't need to say anything. I knew he understood. He knew that he had to work *on* his Body, not just *in* his Body, the way he used to, when he was a runner in high school and college and law school. He knew he had to look at his Body, his Brain, and his Mind as parts of his whole being, with all the parts working in harmony.

"You see, Jon, when you run, you live the life you are supposed to live and fulfill the destiny of what ancient scholastic philosophers called the *actus primus*—the first actuality, the thing that begins a series. The Body is your first actuality; it precedes everything else. Physical exercise—which can be considered the second actuality—connects your Body to your Brain, to your Mind, and even to your Soul.

"But your Soul, Jon, is embodied. We don't know that it can live on its own, after the physical Body dies. All we know, all we are conscious of, is our physical earthly life, in which the Brain, the Mind, and the Soul exist and function within the Body—the *actus primus*."

"That's very interesting," Jon said. "Most people don't put their Body first."

"Indeed, you're right," I responded. "But when you think about it, it is so obvious to do so because we all go through life and recognize and interact with each other with the Body. What is not so obvious is what the Body can teach you about yourself.

"On what may initially seem like a small scale because of its simple nature, running and other hard physical activities can teach you how much you can push yourself and how much you can handle.

"But when you look deeper, you realize that it is not on such a small scale after all that you learn this from physical activity. It is rather on a large scale, in part because the lessons are so blatant and so accessible—you have the opportunity to learn these things about yourself on any day of the week.

"In a very deliberate way, you can find out how much you can handle simply by lacing your shoes and running out the door. You don't need to wait for your resolve to be tested by tragedy, for some illness or accident to happen to you or your loved ones.

"All you need to do is push your Body.

"Seek it out rather than have it inflicted on you. Own it. Take responsibility for it.

"Hard physical exercise can test and reveal your resolve, your courage, your endurance. And you have the choice to learn just how far you can be pushed, how much you can endure, how much you can handle. You can conquer the cowardice in yourself.

"It all starts from the outside. From the physical. From the Body.

"It all starts with working out."

CHAPTER FOUR

Endurance

WHEN YOU CREATE A STRONGER HEART
THAT PUMPS A LOT OF OXYGEN,
YOU CREATE A SOUND BODY.

You're an endurance animal. All humans are. While humans lag well behind other animals when it comes to sprinting—cheetahs, antelopes, horses, foxes, dogs, cats, rabbits, and many other animals can run at much faster speeds than any human—when it comes to endurance, humans run alone. Humans have an unrivaled capacity for endurance running, with no other primates, and few other animals, capable of running long distances.[1] And when it comes to changing your Brain, aerobic endurance exercise is the best type.

Multiple human lineages, including that leading to *Homo sapiens*, evolved in the highlands of Africa at altitudes of 3,300 to 6,600 feet (1,000 to 2,000 meters). Darwin's natural selection would therefore have favored individuals with enhanced aerobic abilities to tolerate the lower oxygen environment of altitude. The physiological traits underlying humans' tolerance to altitude are similar to those associated with greater aerobic endurance. The evolution of human physiology was inherently dependent on efficient oxygen delivery and the development of oxygen-using aerobic metabolism. We needed to use oxygen to survive as a species.

Humans' biological predisposition for endurance may be illustrated by our compelling interest with it. We romanticize the stories of the ancient Greek messenger runner Pheidippides and the Mount Everest climbers, of Ironman triathletes and ultramarathon runners.

When you push the limits of your physical endurance, you find out how much you can endure. And in that discovery, you find out who you really are. Your ability to endure tough situations, to endure stress, to endure suffering—that is what helps you lead a more fulfilling, successful life.

Your heart is one the most important tools for endurance. The ancient Greeks may have been the first to acknowledge the existence of the heart, which they named *kardia*. Aristotle identified the heart as the most important organ of the Body and believed that it was the center of an individual's soul.

The heart is where life lives. How well your cardiovascular system works governs to a large extent how healthy and fit you are, because the cardiovascular system is responsible for delivering oxygen to every cell in your Body, including those in your Brain. Indeed, your Brain cannot function without your heart.

You can't live very well or very long without a strong heart.

Perhaps the most elegant adaptation your Body makes to cardiovascular workouts is an increase in the size of your heart. The enlargement of the left ventricle of your heart causes stronger cardiac contractions and results in a greater stroke volume, which is the amount of blood your heart pumps out with each beat, and a greater cardiac output, which is the amount of blood your heart pumps out each minute. The larger your left ventricle, the more blood it can hold; the more blood it can hold, the more blood (and oxygen) it can pump.

A stronger heart leads to a bigger aerobic engine because the heart's only responsibility is to pump blood that contains oxygen, which is exemplified by the maximum volume of oxygen your Body can consume per minute, called VO_2max.

First measured in humans in the 1920s, VO_2max is the best indicator of your aerobic fitness. When you exercise at your VO_2max, your cardiovascular system is working as hard as it can—your heart rate and stroke volume reach their maximum values, which makes your heart bigger, capable of sending more blood and oxygen throughout your Body, including your Brain. Oxygen flow in the Brain is one of the major factors that stimulates angiogenesis, neurogenesis, and synaptogenesis, creating a sharper, more resilient Mind.

The training of the Body begins with the contractions of the heart and the use of oxygen.

When you create a stronger heart that pumps a lot of oxygen, you create a sound Body.

When you create a sound Body, you create a sound Mind.

The following workouts make your Body aerobically fit and enduring . . . to enable you to live your best life.

RUNNING AND CYCLING VO_2MAX INTERVALS

These VO_2max workouts alternate periods of high-intensity (hard-effort) exercise and low-intensity (easy-effort) recovery. Keep the recovery intervals active to keep oxygen consumption elevated throughout the workout. This helps you reach your VO_2max sooner during each subsequent rep, enabling you to spend more time working at your VO_2max intensity during the workout.

You can do these workouts using your perceived exertion (PE) or a percentage of your maximum heart rate (HR). PE refers to how hard the intensity feels and is based on a scale of 1 (easiest) to 10 (hardest). To determine your maximum heart rate, run 1 mile—four laps of a standard outdoor track—while wearing a chest-strap heart-rate monitor, starting at a comfortable pace and picking it up each lap until you're running all-out over the final lap. Check the heart-rate monitor a few times over the final lap. The highest number you see is your maximum heart rate.

Warm up prior to each workout, starting at a low intensity and progressing to a higher intensity to create a smooth transition from the warm-up to the workout. Begin the workout within a couple of minutes of completing the warm-up.

WORKOUT 1: VO₂MAX INTERVALS
5 reps | 3 minutes | 2 minutes recovery

	Duration (min:sec)	PE	Intensity
Rep #1	3:00	9	>95% max HR
Recovery	2:00	2–3	
Rep #2	3:00	9	>95% max HR
Recovery	2:00	2–3	
Rep #3	3:00	9	>95% max HR
Recovery	2:00	2–3	
Rep #4	3:00	9	>95% max HR
Recovery	2:00	2–3	
Rep #5	3:00	9	>95% max HR

WORKOUT 2: VO₂MAX LADDER
7 reps | 1–4 minutes | 1:1 work:recovery ratio

	Duration (min:sec)	PE	Intensity
Rep #1	1:00	9	>95% max HR
Recovery	1:00	2–3	
Rep #2	1:30	9	>95% max HR
Recovery	1:30	2–3	
Rep #3	2:00	9	>95% max HR
Recovery	2:00	2–3	
Rep #4	2:30	9	>95% max HR
Recovery	2:30	2–3	
Rep #5	3:00	9	>95% max HR
Recovery	3:00	2–3	
Rep #6	3:30	9	>95% max HR
Recovery	3:30	2–3	
Rep #7	4:00	9	>95% max HR

WORKOUT 3: VO₂MAX PYRAMID

9 reps | 1–3 minutes | 1½ minutes recovery

	Duration (min:sec)	PE	Intensity
Rep #1	1:00	9	>95% max HR
Recovery	1:30	2–3	
Rep #2	1:30	9	>95% max HR
Recovery	1:30	2–3	
Rep #3	2:00	9	>95% max HR
Recovery	1:30	2–3	
Rep #4	2:30	9	>95% max HR
Recovery	1:30	2–3	
Rep #5	3:00	9	>95% max HR
Recovery	1:30	2–3	
Rep #6	2:30	9	>95% max HR
Recovery	1:30	2–3	
Rep #7	2:00	9	>95% max HR
Recovery	1:30	2–3	
Rep #8	1:30	9	>95% max HR
Recovery	1:30	2–3	
Rep #9	1:00	9	>95% max HR

WORKOUT 4: VO₂MAX HILLS

5 reps | 3–5 minutes | jog downhill recovery
Find a long, gradual hill that will take you about 3 to 5 minutes to run when you're pushing the pace. Jog slowly back down the hill to recover after each rep.

	Duration (min)	PE	Intensity
Rep #1	3:00–5:00	9	>95% max HR
Recovery	jog downhill	2–3	
Rep #2	3:00–5:00	9	>95% max HR
Recovery	jog downhill	2–3	
Rep #3	3:00–5:00	9	>95% max HR
Recovery	jog downhill	2–3	
Rep #4	3:00–5:00	9	>95% max HR
Recovery	jog downhill	2–3	
Rep #5	3:00–5:00	9	>95% max HR
Recovery	jog downhill	2–3	

RUNNING AND CYCLING TEMPO WORKOUTS

Another important factor of endurance is the lactate threshold, which, technically speaking, is the highest intensity above which lactate quickly accumulates in your muscles and blood. (Since the development of metabolic acidosis begins when the lactate threshold is reached, I often refer to the threshold as the "acidosis threshold" to take the emphasis off the innocuous lactate and place it on the fatigue-inducing acidosis, which is the physiological marker of interest.)

The acidosis threshold demarcates the transition between exercise that is purely aerobic (uses oxygen) and exercise that includes significant anaerobic (oxygen-independent) metabolism. The intensity (speed) at the acidosis threshold is the highest intensity that you can sustain exclusively by aerobic means. If VO_2max represents the size of your aerobic engine, the acidosis threshold represents the fraction or percentage of that engine that you can sustain. Practically speaking, a high acidosis threshold means you have strong endurance. Working out at a higher aerobic "tempo" enhances your Body's and Mind's ability to endure a higher intensity.

Tempo workouts are comfortably hard, at the upper end of being purely aerobic. You can do these workouts using your PE or a percentage of your maximum HR. Warm up prior to each workout, starting at a low intensity and progressing to the intensity at which you will do the workout to create a smooth transition from the warm-up to the workout. Begin the workout within a couple of minutes of completing the warm-up.

WORKOUT 5: TEMPO INTERVALS
5 reps | 5 minutes | 1 minute recovery

	Duration (min)	PE	Intensity
Rep #1	5:00	7–8	80–85% max HR
Recovery	1:00	2–3	
Rep #2	5:00	7–8	80–85% max HR
Recovery	1:00	2–3	
Rep #3	5:00	7–8	80–85% max HR
Recovery	1:00	2–3	
Rep #4	5:00	7–8	80–85% max HR
Recovery	1:00	2–3	
Rep #5	5:00	7–8	80–85% max HR

WORKOUT 6: TEMPO RUN OR RIDE
20–30 minutes
Run or ride continuously at tempo effort. Keep the intensity as steady as possible, with little to no fluctuation.

Duration (min)	PE	Intensity
20–30	7–8	80–85% max HR

WORKOUT 7: TEMPO LONG RUN OR RIDE
Tempo segments should be at 7–8 PE and 80–85% max HR.

Option 1	20 min tempo + 60 min easy
Option 2	60 min easy + 20 min tempo
Option 3	30 min easy + 15 min tempo + 30 min easy + 15 min tempo

Workout 8: Cross-Country Skiing

Cross-country skiing tops the list of best aerobic workouts. It uses most of the muscles of your Body, which increases the demand and use of oxygen. Olympic cross-country skiers are the best human endurance athletes on the planet, with the highest stroke volume (greater than 200 milliliters), cardiac output (in excess of 40 liters per minute), and VO_2max (at least 85 milliliters of oxygen per kilogram of Body weight per minute).[2]

Cross-country skiing outside is a breathtaking experience, both figuratively and literally, especially if you're at altitude. Not many activities are more exhausting yet invigorating than skiing across a blanket of white earth in the middle of nowhere. Explore your surroundings for a couple hours on your skis with the classical style or skating style.

If you don't have access to snow or ski equipment, try roller skiing or rollerblading with ski poles on a flat bike path, or use a cross-country skiing machine in the gym, such as a NordicTrack. If indoors on a guided machine, try pushing the pace with one of the VO_2max interval workouts in this chapter.

Workout 9: Hiking

Hiking may be one of the most underrated forms of endurance exercise. The combination of physical activity and the outdoor environment has a synergistic effect on mood. Research on hiking in the mountains has shown that it causes greater pleasure with less perceived fatigue compared to walking on a treadmill up a similar incline, despite a slightly greater physical stress (as measured by heart rate) while hiking.[3] Research has offered compelling evidence that there is a psychological benefit to exercising in nature, leading to decreased activity in the subgenual prefrontal cortex of the Brain, a region involved in emotional regulation and reward mechanisms, which is more active when individuals are sad and are negatively self-reflective.[4]

To train your Body and your Brain, choose a hike that's challenging, with large variations in altitude. Better yet, go on a several-day hiking trip. That's what Jamie Ash did.

Hiking in Utah, Jamie discovered, was movement for the pleasure of it. "The experience of walking through that landscape—towering red canyon walls rising 600, 800, 1,000 feet, painted with streaks of black varnish deposited over thousands of years, deep sapphire sky above, and electric yellow cottonwood leaves—shifts something in me," she says. "The visual beauty of the place is astounding, but the experience of spending day after day moving, walking, breathing deeply is equally transformational.

"Hiking alone gives me access to a kind of forest quiet: the gurgle of water running over rocks and fallen branches, the hammering of woodpeckers making themselves a roost in a tree, the wind blowing through pine boughs, sometimes soft and gentle, sometimes harsh and ferocious. It's full of physical challenges that I have come to love.

"When I hike in the Columbine-Hondo Wilderness near my home in New Mexico, which climbs to over 12,000 feet of altitude, there's lots of walking uphill, which is never easy. It involves breathing hard, working my muscles, and the determination to get up high. Then there's a big payoff as I look down from a ridge or a summit to the mesas below or across the undulating ridges of mountains. It keeps me emotionally grounded."

CHAPTER FIVE

Strength

WHEN YOU CREATE STRONGER MUSCLES, YOU CREATE A SOUND BODY.

ON PLAYGROUNDS ACROSS THE COUNTRY, ECHOES OF THE phrase, "I bet my muscles are bigger than your muscles" can be heard, as children compare the size of their biceps and show them off to others during recess. School cafeterias turn into venues for arm wrestling, where kids challenge one another at the lunch table, the winner getting his opponent's sandwich. Even children are fascinated with big, strong muscles.

In the early days of physical education, the strength of a muscle garnered all the attention. Tests of muscular strength have existed since at least the time of the ancient Olympics, when athletes were required to lift a ball of iron in order to qualify. In 1873, Dudley Sargent, MD, a pioneer in physical education, initiated strength testing at Harvard University. It has since become an important tool in evaluating muscle characteristics.

Apart from thinking, every human movement requires a muscle action, called a *contraction*. For the discovery that muscles are the organs of voluntary movements, we must go all the way back to 131 to 201 AD and the Greek physician Aelius Galenus, known as Galen. His detailed dissection of the muscles of animals was considered the first attempt at establishing a science of muscles. Early in the second century, he was the first to observe that muscles work in contracting pairs and proposed that muscles pull rather than push.

Many years later, in 1543, Flemish anatomist and physician Andreas Vesalius, author of one of the most influential books on human anatomy, *De Humani Corporis Fabrica Libri Septem* (*On the Fabric of the Human Body*), described the position of each muscle of the Body, with information on its operation, and discovered that the ability of a muscle to contract resides in the muscle itself.

During the mid-eighteenth century, Swiss anatomist and physiologist Albrecht von Haller suggested that the ability to contract is not something that is learned, but rather is an innate property of muscle. Experiments during that era demonstrated that a muscle retains its ability to contract even after death and that contraction of a muscle could be provoked by mechanical, thermal, chemical, or electrical stimuli. The electrical stimuli come from your Brain.

Muscle contraction begins with your nerves. Your central nervous system sends a signal to a neural cell called a *motor neuron*, which integrates with your muscle fibers. Under the action of a neurotransmitter called *acetylcholine*, the signal, called an *action potential*, propagates deep inside your muscle fibers, causing the release of calcium from its storage site and triggering muscle contraction by the complex interaction of specific microscopic proteins.

In 1957, Nobel Prize winner Andrew Huxley from England discovered how those microscopic proteins—actin and myosin—interact. Myosin, which looks like an oar with its paddle at an angle, attaches to actin, which looks like two strings of pearls twisted together. The paddle portion of myosin, which contains the muscles' energy currency that you learned about in high school biology class—ATP—binds to actin, and when ATP is broken down, the paddle portion of myosin pulls the actin so that actin slides past myosin. The mechanism is much like the movement of a rowboat's oars, except that the water (actin) moves past the stationary boat (myosin). This movement happens among millions of actin and myosin proteins within each muscle fiber, with all the actin proteins from opposing sides moving closer together, causing the entire muscle to shorten.

The more actin and myosin proteins inside your muscles, the larger the muscles and the more force they can generate. A boat with eight oars stroking the water is stronger and more powerful than a boat with two.

From the time you were a kid, you knew that bigger muscles are stronger muscles. However, when your Brain gets involved, muscles get stronger even without getting bigger. If you contract your muscles against a heavy enough resistance such that their ability to generate force is challenged, your central nervous system increases the muscles' force by increasing the frequency with which it electrically stimulates motor units (a collection of muscle fibers connected to a single motor neuron) and by recruiting more and larger motor units. In fact, the role your Brain plays in muscle strength is the dominant way your Body gets stronger when you begin working out.

Your Brain regulates a muscle's force in two ways. One way is by recruiting motor units at different frequencies. The frequency of recruitment stimulation is the repeated quickness with which the neuron sends a signal down the axon of the neuron and releases the neurotransmitter acetylcholine into the synapse, which turns the signal into an action potential. The force exerted by each muscle fiber of the motor unit will first increase and then decrease, a response called a *twitch*. Since muscle fibers do not have a latency (rest) period, a second action potential may produce a fiber contraction before the first twitch has subsided. When your Brain increases the frequency of stimulation, a number of action potentials occur in rapid succession, and the resulting twitches are added together, creating a greater force. The higher the frequency of stimulation, the more force is produced, up to a level at which fibers contract tetanically and further increases in the stimulation frequency don't cause a corresponding increase in muscular force.[1] The second way your Brain regulates muscle force is by recruiting an increasingly larger number of motor units. When you lightly contract a muscle, like to pick up a pen from the ground, only a few, small motor units are initially activated. To increase muscular force so that you can pick up a heavy dumbbell from the ground, your Brain recruits progressively larger motor units.

To make your Body strong, your muscles need to produce as much force as possible—and that can happen only if your muscles contract against a heavy resistance.

The training of the Body begins with strong contractions of your muscles.

When you create stronger muscles, you create a sound Body.

When you create a sound Body, you create a sound Mind.

The following workouts make your Body strong and resilient . . . to enable you to live your best life.

WORKOUT 1: FRONT SQUAT
3 sets | 5 reps | 2 minutes rest
Stand in front of a barbell on a squat rack, with the barbell at chest level. Put enough weight on the barbell to fatigue you in 5 reps. Grab the bar with an overhand grip with your hands slightly wider than shoulder-width apart. With your feet shoulder-width or slightly greater than shoulder-width apart, step close to the bar and squat down so that the barbell touches the top of your chest

and front of your shoulders. While gripping the barbell, point your elbows forward and up as high as you can. Stand up to lift the barbell off the rack, keeping your elbows high. The barbell should be resting at the base of your fingers at the knuckles. Step back slightly away from the squat rack. With your back straight, bend your knees and squat down until your thighs are parallel to the ground. Push against the ground to stand up. Repeat for 5 reps.

WORKOUT 2: DEADLIFT
3 sets | 5 reps | 2 minutes rest
Stand in front of a barbell on the ground with feet shoulder-width apart and the front half of your feet under the barbell. Put enough weight on the barbell to fatigue you in 5 reps. With your back straight, squat down and grab the bar with hands shoulder-width apart, one hand with an overhand grip and the other hand with an underhand grip. Keep your back straight, squeeze the bar, and brace your core by keeping your abdominal muscles tight. Stand up by pushing your legs through the ground. Slowly lower the bar by squatting down. Repeat for 5 reps.

WORKOUT 3: TIRE FLIPS
3 sets | 5 reps | 3 minutes recovery
Stand in front of a heavy, oversized tire. Stare it down. Keeping your back straight, bend your knees and lower your hips to squat down to the level of the tire. Grab the tire with both hands with an underhand grip about shoulder-width apart. Keeping your arms stiff and back straight, explosively push against the ground to lift the tire and stand up. Once you have stood up, drive the tire forward and rotate your hands from an underhand grip to overhand grip to prepare to push the tire. Push the tire over by extending your arms. Repeat for 5 reps.

WORKOUT 4: KETTLEBELL CIRCUIT

7 exercises | 10 reps | 3 circuits | 2 minutes recovery

Move immediately from one exercise to the next and recover for 2 minutes before repeating circuit. Select a kettlebell weight that will make you fatigued after 10 reps of each exercise.

	Reps
Kettlebell Swings	10 each arm
Kettlebell Push-Ups with Row	10
Kettlebell Deadlift	10
Kettlebell Russian Twist	10 each side
Kettlebell Goblet Squat	10
Kettlebell Row	10
Kettlebell Squat to Military Press	10

EXERCISE INSTRUCTIONS

Kettlebell Swings

Stand with feet slightly wider than shoulder-width apart. Grab the handle of the kettlebell with your right hand and arm positioned in front of your Body. Bend your knees and drive your hips back as you swing the kettlebell between your legs. Explosively drive your hips forward while swinging the kettlebell upward until your arm is parallel to the ground. Swing the kettlebell back down to the starting position and quickly transfer it to your left hand as it passes through your legs. Repeat the swing with your left arm and continue alternating hands for 10 reps with each arm.

Kettlebell Push-Ups with Row

Kneel on the ground, grabbing the handle of a kettlebell in each hand, and place the kettlebells shoulder-width apart. Assume a standard push-up position with your legs off the ground so that only your toes are touching the ground. Keep your back straight. Bend your arms to lower yourself down until your chest meets the level of your hands. Push yourself back up until your arms are straight and add an upright row after completing each push-up by using your shoulder muscles to lift the right kettlebell a few inches off the ground. Lower the kettlebell back to the ground, do another push-up, and do an upright row with your left arm. Repeat for 10 reps. The exercise can be modified by placing your knees on the ground, flexed to 90 degrees with your ankles crossed.

Kettlebell Deadlift
Stand with feet slightly greater than shoulder-width apart and the kettlebell between your feet. Keeping your back straight, bend into a quarter squat and grab the handle of the kettlebell with both hands. Stand up, keeping your legs straight. Lower the kettlebell until just before it touches the ground and repeat for 10 reps.

Kettlebell Russian Twist
Sit on the ground in a laid-back position, leaning back with your torso, knees bent, and feet flat on the ground or hanging in the air. Hold the kettlebell with both hands in front of your chest. Twist your torso as far as you can to your left side. Hold this position for a brief moment and then twist your torso to your right side. Continue to twist to your left and right sides for 10 reps each side.

Kettlebell Goblet Squat
Stand with feet wider than shoulder-width apart and hold the kettlebell with both hands in front of your chest, keeping your elbows close to your Body. Keeping your back straight, bend your knees and squat down until your thighs are parallel or lower than parallel to the ground. Stand up and repeat for 10 reps.

Kettlebell Row
Grab two kettlebells and stand with feet shoulder-width apart with knees slightly bent. Bend over at the waist. Pull the kettlebells toward your stomach, keeping your back straight and elbows close to your Body. Lower the kettlebells and repeat for 10 reps.

Kettlebell Squat to Military Press

Stand with feet shoulder-width or slightly wider than shoulder-width apart with a kettlebell in each hand and arms fully extended down at your sides with palms facing the side of your legs. Keeping your back straight, bend your knees and squat down until your thighs are parallel to the ground (the kettlebells will be close to touching the ground). Push against the ground to stand up as you lift the kettlebells to shoulder height with elbows pointing down. As you reach the standing position, push the kettlebells upward until your arms are fully extended above your head. Slowly lower the kettlebells to the starting position and repeat for 10 reps.

WORKOUT 5: OBSTACLE COURSE

Imagine running over rough terrain while scaling walls, climbing ropes, and crawling through mud. Obstacle-course workouts test your overall athletic ability, including strength, endurance, and muscle power. The complex movements and changing skills throughout the workout also challenge your Brain. Perhaps the most well-known obstacle-course competitions are Spartan races, which vary in difficulty and distance, from 3 miles to a marathon.

Find a public obstacle course near you, try this simulation workout, or create your own. Run on grass, dirt, or rugged terrain. Move immediately from one exercise to the next.

	Time/Reps
Run	5–10 min
Burpees	10–20
Run	5–10 min
Monkey Bars	swing from one end to other
Run	5–10 min
Fence Climb	climb over & back
Run	5–10 min
Rope Climb	climb up & down
Run	5–10 min
Chin-Ups or Pull-Ups	10

WORKOUT 6: ROCK CLIMBING

Rock climbing is a highly dynamic condition—much like life—with many angles, handholds, footholds, and choices of which paths to navigate. It's great for building dynamic strength, balance, and coordination. Research has shown that dynamic hanging exercises (e.g., pull-ups) cause more fatigue in the arm muscles than does static hanging exercises.[2]

If you haven't rock climbed before, start at an indoor rock climbing gym, where the staff offers classes for beginners. Make sure you have the right equipment—shoes, a bag of chalk, and a harness. Once you have trained your skill and increased your confidence, venture outdoors.

To prepare for rock climbing, train your legs with squats and stair climbs, train your arms with pull-ups, and train your hand and finger strength by gripping heavy books by their spine.

WORKOUT 7: STAND-UP PADDLEBOARDING

While stand-up paddleboarding can be a great way to relax on the water while on vacation, with nature all around you, it's also a great workout. Most people can paddleboard even the first time without much practice. The better your skill, however, the better the workout you can achieve. Stand-up paddleboarding significantly increases upper Body strength, core abdominal and back strength, and balance.

To build muscle endurance, go on a 2-hour paddleboarding journey around the bay or on the lake. For muscle strength and power, try a paddleboarding interval workout: Following a 10-minute warm-up, paddle fast for 60 seconds to propel the board through the water faster, recover for 60 seconds, and repeat 10 times.

WORKOUT 8: WHITEWATER KAYAKING

For a tough workout and an adventure at the same time, whitewater kayaking is a great option. It places exceptional demands on the muscles of your entire upper Body, requiring both high aerobic and anaerobic power, while your lower Body stabilizes you inside the kayak. And the unpredictability of the water demands that you stay aware and adapt to quickly changing conditions, which prepares you for the unpredictable moments in your life. If you have never been kayaking before in the open water, take a class to learn the basics.

CHAPTER SIX

Power

WHEN YOU CREATE POWERFUL MUSCLES, YOU CREATE A SOUND BODY.

WHILE MUSCLE STRENGTH MAY HAVE HOGGED THE ATTENTION of many modern early-century athletes, and even those of the much earlier centuries of ancient Greece, muscles can do a lot more than produce force. When your Body's Chief Operating Officer—your Brain—gets involved, muscles also produce power.

To perform various functions throughout your life, muscle power is even more important than muscle strength, especially as you age.

For your Body to be powerful, it must be strong and it must be fast. Power is the product of muscle strength and muscle contraction speed. It is affected by muscle size, the amount and activity of fast-twitch muscle fibers, and how quickly your Brain sends signals to your muscle fibers to contract. With inactivity and with age, you lose fast-twitch muscle fibers, and the ones you still have get smaller.

To make your muscles powerful, they need to produce as much force as possible as quickly as possible—and that can happen only if your muscles contract quickly.

The training of the Body begins with quick contractions of your muscles.

When you create powerful muscles, you create a sound Body. When you create a sound Body, you create a sound Mind.

The following workouts make your Body powerful . . . to enable you to live your best life.

RUNNING AND CYCLING SPRINT WORKOUTS

These sprint interval workouts alternate periods of fast effort and easy effort recovery. The fast efforts should feel like sprinting, but not so fast that you can't repeat the same intensity after the short recovery. Keep the recovery intervals active. All the workouts are based on time, although a couple of running workouts are based on distance if you have access to a track.

Warm up prior to each workout, starting at a low intensity and progressing to a higher intensity to create a smooth transition from the warm-up to the workout. For example, warm up for 10 minutes at a low intensity, followed by a few bursts at a high intensity for 10 seconds to prime your muscles for the intensity of the workout. Take enough time to recover between each burst since these bursts are not part of the workout and shouldn't cause fatigue; they are only meant to prepare your Body for the intensity of the workout. Begin the workout within a couple of minutes of completing the warm-up.

WORKOUT 1: SPRINT 10 x 10
10 reps | 10 seconds | 30 seconds recovery

	Duration (sec)	Intensity
Rep #1	10	fast
Recovery	30	easy jog or cycle
Rep #2	10	fast
Recovery	30	easy jog or cycle
Rep #3	10	fast
Recovery	30	easy jog or cycle
Rep #4	10	fast
Recovery	30	easy jog or cycle
Rep #5	10	fast
Recovery	30	easy jog or cycle
Rep #6	10	fast
Recovery	30	easy jog or cycle
Rep #7	10	fast
Recovery	30	easy jog or cycle
Rep #8	10	fast
Recovery	30	easy jog or cycle
Rep #9	10	fast
Recovery	30	easy jog or cycle
Rep #10	10	fast

Workout 2: Sprint 10 x 30
10 reps | 30 seconds | 1 minute recovery

	Duration (min:sec)	Intensity
Rep #1	:30	fast
Recovery	1:00	easy jog or cycle
Rep #2	:30	fast
Recovery	1:00	easy jog or cycle
Rep #3	:30	fast
Recovery	1:00	easy jog or cycle
Rep #4	:30	fast
Recovery	1:00	easy jog or cycle
Rep #5	:30	fast
Recovery	1:00	easy jog or cycle
Rep #6	:30	fast
Recovery	1:00	easy jog or cycle
Rep #7	:30	fast
Recovery	1:00	easy jog or cycle
Rep #8	:30	fast
Recovery	1:00	easy jog or cycle
Rep #9	:30	fast
Recovery	1:00	easy jog or cycle
Rep #10	:30	fast

Workout 3: Sprint 10 x 1
10 reps | 1 minute | 2 minutes recovery

	Duration (min)	Intensity
Rep #1	1:00	fast
Recovery	2:00	easy jog or cycle
Rep #2	1:00	fast
Recovery	2:00	easy jog or cycle
Rep #3	1:00	fast
Recovery	2:00	easy jog or cycle
Rep #4	1:00	fast
Recovery	2:00	easy jog or cycle
Rep #5	1:00	fast
Recovery	2:00	easy jog or cycle
Rep #6	1:00	fast
Recovery	2:00	easy jog or cycle
Rep #7	1:00	fast
Recovery	2:00	easy jog or cycle
Rep #8	1:00	fast
Recovery	2:00	easy jog or cycle
Rep #9	1:00	fast
Recovery	2:00	easy jog or cycle
Rep #10	1:00	fast

WORKOUT 4: SPRINT LADDER
2 sets | 5 reps | 10–50 seconds | 1:2 work:recovery ratio

	Duration (min:sec)	Intensity
Set #1		
Rep #1	:10	fast
Recovery	:20	easy jog or cycle
Rep #2	:20	fast
Recovery	:40	easy jog or cycle
Rep #3	:30	fast
Recovery	1:00	easy jog or cycle
Rep #4	:40	fast
Recovery	1:20	easy jog or cycle
Rep #5	:50	fast
Recovery	1:40	easy jog or cycle
Set #2		
Rep #1	:10	fast
Recovery	:20	easy jog or cycle
Rep #2	:20	fast
Recovery	:40	easy jog or cycle
Rep #3	:30	fast
Recovery	1:00	easy jog or cycle
Rep #4	:40	fast
Recovery	1:20	easy jog or cycle
Rep #5	:50	fast

WORKOUT 5: SPRINT PYRAMID
9 reps | 10–50 seconds | 1:2 work:recovery ratio

	Duration (min:sec)	Intensity
Rep #1	:10	fast
Recovery	:20	easy jog or cycle
Rep #2	:20	fast
Recovery	:40	easy jog or cycle
Rep #3	:30	fast
Recovery	1:00	easy jog or cycle
Rep #4	:40	fast
Recovery	1:20	easy jog or cycle
Rep #5	:50	fast
Recovery	1:40	easy jog or cycle
Rep #6	:40	fast
Recovery	1:20	easy jog or cycle
Rep #7	:30	fast
Recovery	1:00	easy jog or cycle
Rep #8	:20	fast
Recovery	:40	easy jog or cycle
Rep #9	:10	fast

WORKOUT 6: TABATA INTERVALS
8 reps | 20 seconds | 10 seconds recovery
Adapted from Japanese scientist Dr. Izumi Tabata's original research, this workout should be done on a stationary bike. Sprint nearly as fast as you can for each 20-second rep. To do the original workout that bears Tabata's name, do this workout five times per week for six weeks.

	Duration (sec)	Intensity
Rep #1	20	nearly all-out
Recovery	10	easy cycle
Rep #2	20	nearly all-out
Recovery	10	easy cycle
Rep #3	20	nearly all-out
Recovery	10	easy cycle
Rep #4	20	nearly all-out
Recovery	10	easy cycle
Rep #5	20	nearly all-out
Recovery	10	easy cycle
Rep #6	20	nearly all-out
Recovery	10	easy cycle
Rep #7	20	nearly all-out
Recovery	10	easy cycle
Rep #8	20	nearly all-out

WORKOUT 7: 400-METER REPS
6–8 reps | 400 meters | 400 meters jog recovery
Do this workout on a 400-meter outdoor track. Use a stopwatch to time
yourself and try to run all reps in the same time.

	Distance (meters)	Intensity
Rep #1	400	fast
Recovery	400	easy jog
Rep #2	400	fast
Recovery	400	easy jog
Rep #3	400	fast
Recovery	400	easy jog
Rep #4	400	fast
Recovery	400	easy jog
Rep #5	400	fast
Recovery	400	easy jog
Rep #6	400	fast
Recovery	400	easy jog
Rep #7	400	fast
Recovery	400	easy jog
Rep #8	400	fast

WORKOUT 8: 200-METER/400-METER REPS
3 sets | 3 reps | 200–400 meters | 200–400 meters jog recovery
Do this workout on a 400-meter outdoor track. Use a stopwatch to time
yourself and try to run the 400s at the same speed as the 200s (i.e., in
exactly double the time).

	Distance (meters)	Intensity
Set #1		
Rep #1	200	fast
Recovery	200	easy jog
Rep #2	200	fast
Recovery	200	easy jog
Rep #3	400	fast
Recovery	400	easy jog
Set #2		
Rep #1	200	fast
Recovery	200	easy jog
Rep #2	200	fast
Recovery	200	easy jog
Rep #3	400	fast
Recovery	400	easy jog
Set #3		
Rep #1	200	fast
Recovery	200	easy jog
Rep #2	200	fast
Recovery	200	easy jog
Rep #3	400	fast

Workout 9: Hill Sprints
10 reps | 30–60 seconds | jog/walk downhill recovery
For this workout, find a short, steep hill that will take you about 30 to 60 seconds to sprint. Jog slowly or walk back down the hill to recover after each rep.

	Duration (sec)	Intensity
Rep #1	30–60	very fast
Recovery	jog/walk downhill	very easy
Rep #2	30–60	very fast
Recovery	jog/walk downhill	very easy
Rep #3	30–60	very fast
Recovery	jog/walk downhill	very easy
Rep #4	30–60	very fast
Recovery	jog/walk downhill	very easy
Rep #5	30–60	very fast
Recovery	jog/walk downhill	very easy
Rep #6	30–60	very fast
Recovery	jog/walk downhill	very easy
Rep #7	30–60	very fast
Recovery	jog/walk downhill	very easy
Rep #8	30–60	very fast
Recovery	jog/walk downhill	very easy
Rep #9	30–60	very fast
Recovery	jog/walk downhill	very easy
Rep #10	30–60	very fast
Recovery	jog/walk downhill	very easy

Workout 10: Hill Accelerators
8 reps | 40 seconds | jog/walk downhill recovery

Find a short, steep hill that will take you about 30 seconds to sprint. When you get to the top, accelerate for another 10 seconds on the flat ground. Jog slowly or walk back down the hill to recover after each rep.

	Duration (sec)	Intensity
Rep #1	30 + 10	fast
Recovery	jog/walk downhill	easy
Rep #2	30 + 10	fast
Recovery	jog/walk downhill	easy
Rep #3	30 + 10	fast
Recovery	jog/walk downhill	easy
Rep #4	30 + 10	fast
Recovery	jog/walk downhill	easy
Rep #5	30 + 10	fast
Recovery	jog/walk downhill	easy
Rep #6	30 + 10	fast
Recovery	jog/walk downhill	easy
Rep #7	30 + 10	fast
Recovery	jog/walk downhill	easy
Rep #8	30 + 10	fast

Workout 11: Plyometrics (Lower Body)
10 exercises | 3 sets | 10 reps | 2 minutes recovery

Do these plyometric exercises on a soft surface with good footing, like grass, artificial turf, or a yoga mat. Transition immediately from one rep to the next, spending as little time as possible on the ground between reps of hops, bounds, and jumps. Think of your legs like springs and focus on exploding off the ground.

	Reps	Sets	Recovery (min)
Vertical Single-Leg Hops	10	3	2:00
Lateral Double-Leg Hops	10	3	2:00
Lateral Single-Leg Hops	10	3	2:00
Bleacher Stair Hops	10	3	2:00
Alternate-Leg Bounds	10	3	2:00
Broad Jumps	10	3	2:00
Speed Skater Jumps	10	3	2:00
Split Jump Lunges	10	3	2:00
Depth Jumps	10	3	2:00
Platform/Box Jumps	10	3	2:00

EXERCISE INSTRUCTIONS

Vertical Single-Leg Hops

Stand with feet together. Pick your left leg up off the ground. Keeping your right leg straight, hop up and down on the ball of your foot. Repeat for 10 reps before switching to the left leg.

Lateral Double-Leg Hops

Place a cone or other similar-height object on the ground. Stand with feet together about 6 inches to the side of the object. While bending your knees slightly, hop side to side on the balls of your feet over the object. Repeat for 10 reps.

Lateral Single-Leg Hops

Place a cone or other similar-height object on the ground. Stand with feet together about 6 inches to the side of the object. Pick your left leg up off the ground. While bending your knee slightly, hop side to side on the ball of your right foot over the object. Repeat for 10 reps before switching to the left leg.

Bleacher Stair Hops

Stand on your right leg at the bottom of the bleacher steps or flight of stairs. With your leg straight, hop up the stairs like a pogo stick, pushing off the ball of your foot. Repeat for 10 reps before switching to the left leg.

Alternate-Leg Bounds

Leap forward off your left leg. As soon as you land on your right foot, push off the ground to leap forward off your right leg. Swing your arms from your shoulders as you would when you run, exaggerating the range of motion. Continue bounding from one leg to the other for 10 reps.

Broad Jumps

Bend your legs in a squat position with thighs parallel to the ground with plenty of space in front of you. From a deep squat, explode up and forward, jumping as far as you can and landing in a squat position. Repeat for 10 reps.

Speed Skater Jumps

Stand with your feet shoulder-width apart. Bend your knees to lower your Body into a half squat and lean forward slightly from the waist, sticking your butt out. Shift your weight onto your left leg and pick your right leg up off the ground and place it behind your left ankle. Then, hop sideways to your right by pushing with the outside edge of your left foot and land on your right foot, bringing your left leg behind your right ankle. Swing your arms in concert with your legs so that your right arm is forward when your left leg lands and vice versa. Continue hopping from one side to the other for 10 reps with each leg.

Split Jump Lunges

Stand with your feet shoulder-width apart. Step forward about 2 feet with your right leg and lower yourself down into the lunge while keeping your torso upright. Keep your right knee above your toes as you lunge forward and keep your right shin perpendicular to the ground. From this lunge position, jump up into the air with both feet while switching your leg position in midair and land with your left leg forward. Repeat for 10 reps with each leg.

Depth Jumps
Stand on a firm platform or plyometric box about 2 feet tall with your legs shoulder-width apart. Jump onto the ground and land in a squat position with your thighs parallel to the ground and your knees in line with your toes. From this squat position, jump straight up as high as possible. Repeat for 10 reps.

Platform/Box Jumps
Stand in front of a firm platform or plyometric box about 2 feet high in a squat position with your feet shoulder-width apart and knees bent. Jump with two feet onto the platform. As soon as you land, jump into the air and back down to the ground on the other side of the platform. To make the exercise more challenging, jump with one foot at a time. Repeat for 10 reps.

WORKOUT 12: PLYOMETRICS (UPPER BODY)
5 exercises | 3 sets | 10 reps | 2 minutes recovery
Transition immediately from one rep to the next, spending as little time as possible touching the ground or object between reps. Think of your arms like springs and focus on exploding off the object.

	Reps	Sets	Recovery (min)
Medicine Ball Toss	10	3	2:00
Plyometric Push-Ups	10	3	2:00
Volleyball Toss	10	3	2:00
Boxing Punches	10	3	2:00
Depth Push-Ups	10	3	2:00

EXERCISE INSTRUCTIONS

Medicine Ball Toss

Stand with feet shoulder-width apart. Hold an 8- to 10-pound medicine ball with both hands and palms facing away from you. With your knees slightly bent and core tight, throw the medicine ball with two hands from your chest to your partner. Catch the medicine ball with outstretched arms, drawing your arms into your chest in one smooth movement and quickly throw it back to your partner. (If you don't have a partner, throw the medicine ball against a wall.) Repeat for 10 reps.

Plyometric Push-Ups

Assume a standard push-up position, with legs lifted off the ground and back straight. Place your hands slightly greater than shoulder-width apart. Lower yourself down until your chest comes close to the ground and, then, explosively push off the ground, allowing your hands to lift off the ground. Land in the starting push-up position, and immediately complete the next rep. Repeat for 10 reps. The exercise can be modified by clapping your hands together in midair, or by placing your hands on a bench or by placing your knees on the ground and flexed to 90 degrees with ankles crossed.

Volleyball Toss

Stand with feet shoulder-width apart. Hold a volleyball with both hands and palms facing away from you. With your arms bent, toss the volleyball with both hands from your chest straight up into the air like a volleyball pass. "Catch" the volleyball with bent arms, and quickly toss it back up again. Repeat for 10 reps.

Boxing Punches

Stand in front of a punching bag with boxing gloves on, and throw short, compact jabs at the bag, retracting your gloved hand from the bag immediately after making contact. If you have a partner, have your partner wear boxing mitts, and throw short, compact jabs at the mitts. Punch 10 times before punching with the other hand.

Depth Push-Ups

Place two small plyometric boxes or similar raised platforms on the ground about shoulder-width apart. Get into a push-up position, with a hand on each box. Quickly remove your hands from the boxes toward your Body and let them drop down to the ground, with elbows slightly bent. Let your upper Body "fall" until your chest comes close to the ground. Then, immediately and explosively push off the ground, allowing your hands to lift off the ground, and quickly place your hands back onto the boxes. Repeat for 10 reps.

CHAPTER SEVEN

Cognitive Flexibility

WHEN YOU CREATE COGNITIVE FLEXIBILITY, YOU CREATE A SOUND BODY.

AT SOME POINT IN YOUR LIFE, YOU HAVE PROBABLY BEEN ASKED (or even tried) to rub your belly in a circular motion with one hand while tapping your head with your other hand. Not so easy, is it? The reason it's not so easy is because performing those motions simultaneously requires *cognitive flexibility*: Your Brain must think, plan, and execute two asymmetric movements at once.

Exercise that requires elements of cognitive flexibility (e.g., thought, planning, concentration, problem-solving, working memory, and/or inhibitory control) improves coordination and agility of your Body and your Brain. For example, a football quarterback's Brain must deal with constantly changing situations. He must mentally work with lots of information, remember complex movement sequences, react to external stimuli while moving around the football field, process other players' movements and make quick decisions based on them, plan the trajectory of the football to reach its destination in a wide receiver's hands 30 yards away, use working memory to compare the present situation to past situations to predict what is likely to happen next, inhibit attending to distractions, and focus attention on the specific task.

That's a lot to do all at once. But your Brain can do it if you train it to do it, using your Body as the training tool.

The training of the Body begins with cognitive flexibility workouts.

When you create cognitive flexibility, you create a sound Body, with millions of neurons and synapses buzzing with activity inside your Brain that can think on its feet.

When you create a sound Body, you create a sound Mind capable of making quick, accurate assessments of situations and making smart, precise decisions.

The following workouts make your Body coordinated and agile, your Brain flexible, and your Mind sharp . . . to enable you to live your best life.

WORKOUT 1: SPRINT/BODY-WEIGHT CIRCUIT

12 exercises | 30 sec/10–15 reps | 1–2 circuits | 2 minutes recovery
This complex circuit that constantly changes the movement sequences sprint running with a lower-Body exercise, upper-Body exercise, and core exercise for a total-Body and Brain workout. Move immediately from one exercise to the next and recover for 2 minutes if you do the circuit twice. Make the sprint fast and challenging, but not all-out.

	Time/Reps
Sprint	30 sec
Squat Jumps	10–15
Push-Ups	10–15
Pike Crunches	10–15
Sprint	30 sec
Squat Side Steps	10–15 each side
Superman	10–15
V-Sit	10–15
Sprint	30 sec
Mountain Climbers	10–15 each leg
Triceps Dips	10–15
Russian Twists	10–15

WORKOUT 2: BASKETBALL SPRINT AND SHOOT CIRCUIT
4 sprints | 6 shots | 5 circuits | 2 minutes recovery

This workout forces you to focus and aim when breathing hard. From the baseline of a basketball court, sprint the length of the court to the opposite baseline and back, to the opposite free-throw line and back, to the mid-court line and back, and to the near free-throw line and back. When you get to each free-throw line, take three shots. To challenge your Brain even more, dribble a basketball while sprinting and take a lay-up shot at each end of the court. You can also run and take shots from different parts of the court. Recover for 2 minutes before repeating the circuit.

WORKOUT 3: SPRINT INTERVALS WITH DIRECTION CHANGE
4 sprints | 3 direction changes | 10 circuits | 1 minute recovery

This workout improves your acceleration, agility, and ability to react quickly. Using cones, set up a large square on a grass field. Sprint straight ahead for 3 seconds to the first cone, side shuffle quickly to the next cone, turn around and sprint to the next cone, and side shuffle quickly to the final cone. Focus on moving your feet as fast as possible. Recover for 1 minute before repeating the circuit. For variety, set up the cones in different patterns (diamond, triangle, octagon, etc.).

WORKOUT 4: AGILITY LADDER DRILLS CIRCUIT
6 exercises | 10 reps | 3 circuits | 1 minute recovery

Place an agility ladder vertically on the ground. For each exercise, move your feet as fast and controlled as you can. Move immediately from one exercise to the next and recover for 1 minute between circuits.

	Reps
Forward High Knees	10
Lateral High Knees	10
Forward-Side Hops	10
Ins-Outs	10
Slalom Hops	10
Lateral Split Jump Lunges	10

Exercise Instructions
Forward High Knees
Stand facing forward in front of the ladder. Run with high knees forward through the ladder, placing a foot in each box. When you get to the end of the ladder, sprint for 3 seconds.

Lateral High Knees
Stand in front of the ladder, with the ladder to your left. Run sideways to your left with high knees through the ladder, placing a foot in each box. When you get to the end of the ladder, turn forward and sprint for 3 seconds.

Forward-Side Hops
Stand on the right side of the ladder, facing forward. Hop laterally into the first box with your left foot first, immediately followed by your right foot. Push off to the side with your right foot and hop outside to the left of the box with your left foot, then immediately push off your left foot and hop back into the box with your right foot. Push off your right foot and hop forward with your left foot into the next box. Push off to the side with your left foot and hop outside to the right of the box with your right foot, then immediately push off your right foot and hop back into box with your left foot. Repeat the forward-side hopping pattern for the length of the ladder. When you get to the end of the ladder, sprint for 3 seconds.

Ins-Outs
Stand facing forward in front of the ladder. Hop into the first box with your left foot first, immediately followed by your right foot. With your left foot, hop outside to the left of the second box, then immediately hop outside the second box with your right foot. Hop back into the third box with your left foot first, followed by your right foot. Repeat this in-out hopping pattern for the length of the ladder. When you get to the end of the ladder, sprint for 3 seconds.

Slalom Hops

Start with your right foot inside the first box and your left foot outside the box. With both feet, hop to the next box and land with your left foot inside the box and your right foot outside the box. Then, hop to the next box, landing with your right foot in the box and left foot outside the box. Hop the length of the ladder, alternating feet landing inside and outside the box. Keep your legs slightly bent the whole time, like a slalom skier. When you get to the end of the ladder, sprint for 3 seconds.

Lateral Split Jump Lunges

Stand to the side of the ladder, facing the first box. Step forward with your right leg, place your foot into the box, and lower yourself down into the lunge while keeping your torso upright. Keep your right knee above your toes as you lunge forward and keep your right shin perpendicular to the ground. From this lunge position, jump up into the air with both feet while switching your leg position in midair and land with your left foot forward in the next box. Jump up again and land with your right foot in the same box. Repeat the pattern until you reach the end of the ladder, and then sprint for 3 seconds.

WORKOUT 5: RACQUETBALL

The fast-moving game of racquetball trains your Brain as well as your Body. It includes hand-eye coordination, constant and quick changes of direction, quick decision-making, judgment of where the ball is going to be, coordination to hit the ball with the racquet, and judgment of the angles to both plan where to hit the ball and react to it as it bounces against the walls and onto the court. Find a friend who, like you, wants to create a sound Body to create a sound Mind, and go to a gym with racquetball courts.

WORKOUT 6: SOCCER

The unnatural foot-eye coordination of soccer challenges your Brain in a unique way. Like racquetball, soccer is an open-skilled activity, which means you have to react dynamically to a constantly changing, unpredictable environment. Soccer also includes a lot of running, especially for the forward and midfielder positions. Kicking, running while controlling the ball with your feet, passing the ball to a teammate, aiming shots on goal, and defending against players of the opposing team, all with your feet, are great for improving coordination, balance, agility, and quickness. And that means it's also great for your Brain. Several studies have shown positive relationships between basic cognitive functions and physical soccer skills.[1] So take a ball to the park with a friend and practice your soccer skills, gather several friends for a pick-up game, or join a recreational team to play in a league.

WORKOUT 7: ICE HOCKEY

If you can ice skate, the fast-paced and physical game of ice hockey requires both hand-eye and foot-eye coordination. Moving on a 3-millimeter-wide steel blade on a sheet of ice while holding a long stick to shoot a rubber puck, ice hockey challenges your Body and Brain in multiple ways. Physically, it includes both aerobic and anaerobic elements, quickness, balance, coordination, agility, and stick-handling skill. Cognitively, it includes quick decision-making, direction changes, reading other players' movements and planning around them, prediction of puck location, estimation of how hard and in what direction to shoot the puck to pass it to another player, and accurate aim to shoot the puck into the goal, all while you're skating on ice.

Epilogue

AN ENTIRE YEAR HAD PASSED SINCE MY LAST CONVERSATION with Jon. I was curious to learn what he had been up to and how his life was going.

This time, we didn't meet at his office. We met for a run.

Jon is nearly a decade younger than I, and a much more talented runner. Even with the extra weight he had put on during the years of not running, he was still faster than I. So I had to do my best to keep up.

"How's it going?" I asked him, as we started running just north of downtown Indianapolis along the lush green tree-lined Monon Trail, the paved rail trail named after the popular defunct railroad line connecting Indianapolis and Chicago.

"I'm down 20 pounds since I started running again," he said, without taking a breath.

"That's great!" I exclaimed, secretly worried that he may be fit enough to push the pace.

"I feel like a million bucks!" he said. "My life is so much better. I have a lot more clarity. I feel less stressed at work, and I don't bring my work home with me anymore."

My heart swelled with emotion. I was genuinely happy for Jon, in part because I remembered how happy and positive he was years ago when he was running every day, and in part because Jon was beginning to see the great power physical training has to change the three parts of himself—Body, Brain, and Mind—which affects everything he does.

"I may even start racing again once I get back into shape," Jon said.

"Definitely," I said, encouragingly.

"I've been thinking about what you said, about us being animals," Jon said. "You're right. I definitely feel differently when I run and during the rest of the day. I had forgotten what it felt like. It's hard to explain. It's like I feel more *physical*."

"That's a great insight," I responded, smiling to myself.

"There are times in your life that will test you, Jon, that will throw you on your back. But if you remember where you came from, if you remember that you are indeed an animal with biology similar to that of many other animals, then you remember that to live life fully, you must fully live physically. And then, you can train your Body to change your Brain to affect your Mind, connecting the three parts of yourself that create your earthly existence."

Notes

Prologue
1. Taylor, C.R., and Weibel, E.R. Design of the mammalian respiratory system. I. Problem and strategy. *Respiration Physiology*, 44(1):1–10, 1981.
2. Weibel, E.R., Taylor, C.R., and Hoppeler, H. The concept of symmorphosis: A testable hypothesis of structure-function relationship. *Proceedings of the National Academy of Sciences*, 88:10357–10361, 1991.
3. Weibel, E.R. *Symmorphosis: On Form and Function in Shaping Life*. Cambridge, MA: Harvard University Press, 2000.

Chapter 1: Body
1. Hönekopp, J., Rudolph, U., Beier, L., Liebert, A., and Müller, C. Physical attractiveness of face and body as indicators of physical fitness in men. *Evolution and Human Behavior*, 28:106–111, 2007.
2. Postma, E. A relationship between attractiveness and performance in professional cyclists. *Biology Letters*, 10(2):20130966, 2014.
3. Schulte-Hostedde, A.I., Eys, M.A., Emond, M., and Buzdon, M. Sport participation influences perceptions of mate characteristics. *Evolutionary Psychology*, 10(1):78–94, 2012.
4. Hoffmann, M., and Pfeifer, R. The implications of embodiment for behavior and cognition: Animal and robotic case studies. In: Tschacher, W. and Bergomi, C. (Eds.). *The Implications of Embodiment: Cognition and Communication*. Exeter, United Kingdom: Imprint Academic, 31–58, 2012.
5. Barrès, R., Yan, J., Egan, B., Treebak, J.T., Rasmussen, M., Fritz, T., Caidahl, K., Krook, A., O'Gorman, D.J., and Zierath, J.R. Acute exercise remodels promoter methylation in human skeletal muscle. *Cell Metabolism*, 15(3):405–411, 2012.
6. Rönn, T., Volkov, P., Davegårdh, C., Dayeh, T., Hall, E., Olsson, A.H., Nilsson, E., Tornberg, A., Dekker Nitert, M., Eriksson, K.F., Jones, H.A., Groop, L., and Ling, C. A six months exercise intervention influences the genome-

wide DNA methylation pattern in human adipose tissue. *PLOS Genetics*, 9(6):e1003572, 2013.

7. Fernandes, J., Arida, R.M., and Gomez-Pinilla, F. Physical exercise as an epigenetic modulator of brain plasticity and cognition. *Neuroscience and Biobehavioral Reviews*, 80:443–456, 2017.

8. Karp, J.R. *Sexercise: Exercising Your Way to Better Sex*. Pennsauken, NJ: BookBaby, 2020.

9. Booth, F.W., Laye, M.J., and Roberts, M.D. Lifetime sedentary living accelerates some aspects of secondary aging. *Journal of Applied Physiology*, 111(5):1497–1504, 2011.

10. Charansonney, O.L. Physical activity and aging: A life-long story. *Discovery Medicine*, 12(64):177–185, 2011.

11. Batt, S. Human attitudes towards animals in relation to species similarity to humans: A multivariate approach. *Bioscience Horizons*, 2(2):180–190, 2009.

12. Meijer, J.H., and Robbers, Y. Wheel running in the wild. *Proceedings of the Royal Society: Biological Sciences*, 281(1786):20140210, 2014.

13. Cordain, L., Gotshall, R.W., and Eaton, S.B. Evolutionary aspects of exercise. *World Review of Nutrition and Dietetics*, 81:49–60, 1997.

14. Gould, S.J. *The Panda's Thumb: More Reflections in Natural History*. New York: W.W. Norton & Company, 1992.

15. Klein, R.G. *The Human Career: Human Biological and Cultural Origins*. Chicago: University of Chicago Press, 1999.

Chapter 2: Brain

1. Colzato, L.S., Szapora, A., Pannekoek, J.N., and Hommel, B. The impact of physical exercise on convergent and divergent thinking. *Frontiers in Human Neuroscience*, 7:824, 2013.

2. Tomporowski, P.D., and Ellis, N.R. Effects of exercise on cognitive processes: A review. *Psychological Bulletin*, 99(3):338–346, 1986.

3. Oppezzo, M., and Schwartz, D.L. Give your ideas some legs: The positive effect of walking on creative thinking. *Journal of Experimental Psychology: Learning, Memory, and Cognition*, 40(4):1142–1152, 2014.

4. Steinberg, H., Sykes, E.A., Moss, T., Lowery, S., LeBoutillier, N., and Dewey, A. Exercise enhances creativity independently of mood. *British Journal of Sports Medicine*, 31:240–245, 1997.

5. Aberg, M.A., Pedersen, N.L., Toren, K., Svartengren, M., Bäckstrand, B., Johnsson, T., Cooper-Kuhn, C.M., Aberg, N.D., Nilsson, M., and Kuhn, H.G. Cardiovascular fitness is associated with cognition in young adulthood. *Proceedings of the National Academy of Sciences of the United States of America*, 106(49):20906–20911, 2009.

6. Arida R.M., and Teixeira-Machado, L. The contribution of physical exercise to brain resilience. *Frontiers in Behavioral Neuroscience*, 14:626769, 2021.

7. Singh-Manoux, A., Hillsdon, M., Brunner, E., and Marmot, M. Effects of physical activity on cognitive functioning in middle age: Evidence from

the Whitehall II prospective cohort study. *American Journal of Public Health*, 95(12):2252–2258, 2005.

8. Trudeau, F., and Shephard, R.J. Physical education, school physical activity, school sports and academic performance. *International Journal of Behavioral Nutrition and Physical Activity*, 5:10, 2008.

9. Donnelly, J.E., Hillman, C.H., Castelli, D., Etnier, J.L., Lee, S., Tomporowski, P., Lambourne, K., and Szabo-Reed, A.N. Physical activity, fitness, cognitive function, and academic achievement in children: A systematic review. *Medicine and Science in Sports and Exercise*, 48(6):1197–1222, 2016.

10. Immordino-Yang, M.H., and Damasio, A. We feel, therefore we learn: The relevance of affective and social neuroscience to education. *Mind, Brain, and Education*, 1(1):3–10, 2007.

11. Doherty, A., and Miravalles, A.F. Physical activity and cognition: Inseparable in the classroom. *Frontiers in Education*, 4:105, 2019.

12. Clapp, J.F., III. Morphometric and neurodevelopmental outcome at age five years of the offspring of women who continued to exercise regularly throughout pregnancy. *Journal of Pediatrics*, 129(6):856–863, 1996.

13. Esteban-Cornejo, I., Martinez-Gomez, D., Tejero-González, C.M., Izquierdo-Gomez, R., Carbonell-Baeza, A., Castro-Piñero, J., Sallis, J.F., and Veiga, O.L. Maternal physical activity before and during the prenatal period and the offspring's academic performance in youth. The UP&DOWN study. *Journal of Maternal-Fetal Neonatal Medicine*, 29(9):1414–1420, 2015.

14. Arida R.M., and Teixeira-Machado, L. The contribution of physical exercise to brain resilience. *Frontiers in Behavioral Neuroscience*, 14:626769, 2021.

15. Kuusi, P. *This World of Man*. Oxford: Pergamon Press, 1985.

16. Wood, B., and Collard, M. The human genus. *Science*, 284:65–71, 1999.

17. Cobb, S. *Foundations of Neuropsychiatry*. Baltimore: Williams & Wilkins, 1941.

18. Leisman, G., Moustafa, A.A., and Shafir, T. Thinking, walking, talking: Integratory motor and cognitive brain function. *Frontiers in Public Health*, 4:94, 2016.

19. Diamond, A. Close interrelation of motor development and cognitive development and of the cerebellum and prefrontal cortex. *Child Development*, 71(1):44–56, 2000.

20. Kleckner, I.R., Zhang, J., Touroutoglou, A., Chanes, L., Xia, C., Simmons, W.K., Quigley, K.S., Dickerson, B.C., and Feldman Barrett, L. Evidence for a large-scale brain system supporting allostasis and interoception in humans. *Nature Human Behavior*, 1:0069, 2017.

21. Fontes, E.B., Okano, A.H., De Guio, F., Schabort, E.J., Min, L.L., Basset, F.A., Stein, D.J., and Noakes, T.D. Brain activity and perceived exertion during cycling exercise: An fMRI study. *British Journal of Sports Medicine*, 49(8):556–560, 2015.

22. Raichlen, D.A., Bharadwaj, P.K., Fitzhugh, M.C., Haws, K.A., Torre, G.-A., Trouard, T.P., and Alexander, G.E. Differences in resting state functional connectivity between young adult endurance athletes and healthy controls. *Frontiers in Human Neuroscience*, 10:610, 2016.

23. Schmitta, A., Upadhyayb, N., Martina, J.A., Rojasc, S., Strüder, H.K., and Boecker, H. Modulation of distinct intrinsic resting state brain networks by acute exercise bouts of differing intensity. *Brain Plasticity*, 5(1):39–55, 2019.

24. Erickson, K.I., Weinstein, A.M., Sutton, B.P., Prakash, R.S., Voss, M.W., Chaddock, L., Szabo, A.N., Mailey, E.L., White, S.M., Wojcicki, T.R., McAuley, E., and Kramer, A.F. Beyond vascularization: Aerobic fitness is associated with N-acetylaspartate and working memory. *Brain and Behavior*, 2(1):32–41, 2012.

25. Hötting, K., and Röder, B. Beneficial effects of physical exercise on neuroplasticity and cognition. *Neuroscience and Biobehavioral Reviews*, 37:2243–2257, 2013.

26. Di Liegro, C.M., Schiera, G., Proia, P., and Di Liegro, I. Physical activity and brain health. *Genes*, 10(9):720, 2019.

27. Cherup, N., Roberson, K., Potiaumpai, M., Widdowson, K., Jaghab, A.M., Chowdhari, S., Armitage, C., Seeley, A., and Signorile, J. Improvements in cognition and associations with measures of aerobic fitness and muscular power following structured exercise. *Experimental Gerontology*, 112:76–87, 2018.

28. McDaniel, M.A., Einstein, G.O., and Jacoby, L.L. New consideration in aging and memory: The glass may be half full. In: Craik, F.I.M., and Salthouse, T.A. (Eds.). *The Handbook of Aging and Cognition*, New York: Psychology Press, 251–310, 2008.

29. Tivadar, B.K. Physical activity improves cognition: Possible explanations. *Biogerontology*, 18:477–483, 2017.

30. Gregory, M.A., Gill, D.P., and Petrella, R.J. Brain health and exercise in older adults. *Current Sports Medicine Reports*, 12(4):256–271, 2013.

31. Lautenschlager, N.T., Cox, K.L., Flicker, L., Foster, J.K., van Bockxmeer, F.M., Xiao, J., Greenop, K.R., and Almeida, O.P. Effect of physical activity on cognitive function in older adults at risk for Alzheimer disease: A randomized trial. *Journal of the American Medical Association*, 300(9):1027–1037, 2008.

32. Cotman, C.W., and Engesser-Cesar, C. Exercise enhances and protects brain function. *Exercise and Sport Sciences Reviews*, 30(2):75–79, 2002.

33. Raichien, D.A., and Gordon, A.D. Relationship between exercise capacity and brain size in mammals. *PLOS ONE*, 6(6):e20601, 2011.

34. Erickson, K.I., Leckie, R.L., and Weinstein, A.M. Physical activity, fitness, and gray matter volume. *Neurobiology of Aging*, 35(Suppl 2):S20–S28, 2014.

35. Taki, Y., Kinomura, S., Sato, K., Goto, R., Kawashima, R., and Fukuda, H. A longitudinal study of gray matter volume decline with age and modifying factors. *Neurobiology of Aging*, 32(5):907–915, 2011.

36. Yuki, A., Lee, S., Kim, H., Kozakai, R., Ando, F., and Shimokata, H. Relationship between physical activity and brain atrophy progression. *Medicine and Science in Sports and Exercise*, 44(12):2362–2368, 2012.

37. Firth, J., Stubbs, B., Vancampfort, D., Schuch, F., Lagopoulos, J., Rosenbaum, S., and Ward, P.B. Effect of aerobic exercise on hippocampal volume in humans: A systematic review and meta-analysis. *NeuroImage*, 166:230–238, 2018.

38. Erickson, K.I., Leckie, R.L., and Weinstein, A.M. Physical activity, fitness, and gray matter volume. *Neurobiology of Aging*, 35(Suppl 2):S20–S28, 2014.

39. Kilgour, A.H.M., Todd, O.M., and Starr, J.M. A systematic review of the evidence that brain structure is related to muscle structure and their relationship to brain and muscle function in humans over the lifecourse. *BMC Geriatrics*, 14:85, 2014.

40. Atkinson, H.H., Rosano, C., Simonsick, E.M., Williamson, J.D., Davis, C., Ambrosius, W.T., Rapp, S.R., Cesari, M., Newman, A.B., Harris, T.B., Rubin, S.M., Yaffe, K., Satterfield, S., and Kritchevsky, S.B. Cognitive function, gait speed decline, and comorbidities: The health, aging and body composition study. *Journal of Gerontology*, 62A(8):844–850, 2007.

41. Duff, K., Mold, J.W., and Roberts, M.M. Walking speed and global cognition: Results from the OKLAHOMA Study. *Aging, Neuropsychology, and Cognition*, 15(1):31–39, 2008.

42. von Bartheld, C.S., Bahney, J., and Herculano-Houzel, S. The search for true numbers of neurons and glial cells in the human brain: A review of 150 years of cell counting. *The Journal of Comparative Neurology*, 524(18):3865–3895, 2016.

43. Herculano-Houzel, S. *The Human Advantage: A New Understanding of How Our Brain Became Remarkable*. Cambridge, MA: MIT Press, 2016.

44. Ramón y Cajal, S. Translated by May, R.M. *Degeneration and Regeneration of the Nervous System*. London: Oxford University Press, 1928.

45. van Praag, H. Neurogenesis and exercise: Past and future directions. *Neuromolecular Medicine*, 10(2):128–140, 2008.

46. Cassilhas, R.C., Tufik, S., and Túlio de Mello, M. Physical exercise, neuroplasticity, spatial learning and memory. *Cellular and Molecular Life Sciences*, 73(5):975–983, 2016.

47. Hamilton, G.F., and Rhodes, J.S. Exercise regulation of cognitive function and neuroplasticity in the healthy and diseased brain. *Progress in Molecular Biology and Translational Science*, 135:381–406, 2015.

48. Voss, M.W., Nagamatsu, L.S., Liu-Ambrose, T., and Kramer, A.F. Exercise, brain, and cognition across the life span. *Journal of Applied Physiology*, 111:1505–1513, 2011.

49. El-Sayes, J., Harasym, D., Turco, C.V., Locke, M.B., and Nelson, A.J. Exercise-induced neuroplasticity: A mechanistic model and prospects for promoting plasticity. *The Neuroscientist*, 25(1):65–68, 2019.

50. Draganski, B., and May, A. Training-induced structural changes in the adult human brain. *Behavioural Brain Research*, 192:137–142, 2008.

51. Altman, J. Are new neurons formed in the brains of adult mammals? *Science*, 135(3509):1127–1128, 1962.

52. Altman, J., and Das, G.D. Autoradiographic and histological evidence of postnatal hippocampal neurogenesis in rats. *Journal of Comparative Neurology*, 124(3):319–335, 1965.

53. Eriksson, P.S., Perfilieva, E., Björk-Eriksson, T., Alborn, A.M., Nordborg, C., Peterson, D.A., and Gage, F.H. Neurogenesis in the adult human hippocampus. *Nature Medicine*, 4(11):1313–1317, 1998.

54. Rhodes, J.S., van Praag, H., Jeffrey, S., Girard, I., Mitchell, G.S., Garland, T., Jr., and Gage, F.H. Exercise increases hippocampal neurogenesis to high levels but does not improve spatial learning in mice bred for increased voluntary wheel running. *Behavioral Neuroscience*, 117(5):1006–1016, 2003.

55. Dostes, S., Dubreucq, S., Ladevèze, E., Marsicano, G., Abrous, D.N., Francis Chaouloff, F., and Koehl, M. Running per se stimulates the dendritic arbor of newborn dentate granule cells in mouse hippocampus in a duration-dependent manner. *Hippocampus*, 26(3):282–288, 2016.

56. Vilela, T.C., Muller, A.P., Damiani, A.P., Macan, T.P., da Silva, S., Canteiro, P.B., de Sena Casagrande, A., Pedroso, G.D.S., Nesi, R.T., de Andrade, V.M., and de Pinho, R.A. Strength and aerobic exercises improve spatial memory in aging rats through stimulating distinct neuroplasticity mechanisms. *Molecular Neurobiology*, 54(10):7928–7937, 2017.

57. Christie, B.R., Eadie, B.D., Kannangara, T.S., Robillard, J.M., Shin, J., and Titterness, A.K. Exercising our brains: How physical activity impacts synaptic plasticity in the dentate gyrus. *Neuromolecular Medicine*, 10(2):47–58, 2008.

58. Clark, P.J., Kohman, R.A., Miller, D.S., Bhattacharya, T.K., Brzezinska, W.J., and Rhodes, J.S. Genetic influences on exercise-induced adult hippocampal neurogenesis across 12 divergent mouse strains. *Genes, Brain and Behavior*, 10:345–353, 2011.

59. Ferreira, A.F., Real, C.C., Rodrigues, A.C., Alves, A.S., and Britto, L.R. Moderate exercise changes synaptic and cytoskeletal proteins in motor regions of the rat brain. *Brain Research*, 1361:31–42, 2010.

60. Wrann, C.D., White, J.P., Salogiannnis, J., Laznik-Bogoslavski, D., Wu, J., Ma, D., Lin, J.D., Greenberg, M.E., and Spiegelman, B.M. Exercise induces hippocampal BDNF through a PGC-1α/FNDC5 pathway. *Cell Metabolism*, 18(5):649–659, 2013.

61. Szuhany, K.L., Bugatti, M., and Otto, M.W. A meta-analytic review of the effects of exercise on brain-derived neurotrophic factor. *Journal of Psychiatric Research*, 60:56–64, 2015.

62. Liu, P.Z., and Nusslock, R. Exercise-mediated neurogenesis in the hippocampus via BDNF. *Frontiers in Neuroscience*, 12:52, 2018.

63. Marosi, K., and Mattson, M.P. BDNF mediates adaptive brain and body responses to energetic challenges. *Trends in Endocrinology and Metabolism*, 25(2):89–98, 2014.

64. Egginton, S. In vivo models of muscle angiogenesis. *Methods in Molecular Biology*, 1430:355–373, 2016.

65. Hoier, B., and Hellsten, Y. Exercise-induced capillary growth in human skeletal muscle and the dynamics of VEGF. *Microcirculation*, 21:301–314, 2014.

66. El-Sayes, J., Harasym, D., Turco, C.V., Locke, M.B., and Nelson, A.J. Exercise-induced neuroplasticity: A mechanistic model and prospects for promoting plasticity. *The Neuroscientist*, 25(1):65–68, 2019.

67. Egginton, S. Invited review: Activity-induced angiogenesis. *Pflügers Archiv: European Journal of Physiology*, 457(5):963–977, 2009.

68. Isaacs, K.R., Anderson, B.J., Alcantara, A.A., Black, J.E., and Greenough, W.T. Exercise and the brain: Angiogenesis in the adult rat cerebellum after vigorous physical activity and motor skill learning. *Journal of Cerebral Blood Flow and Metabolism*, 12:110–119, 1992.

69. Kerr, A.L., Steuer, E.L., Pochtarev, V., and Swain, R.A. Angiogenesis but not neurogenesis is critical for normal learning and memory acquisition. *Neuroscience*, 171:214–226, 2010.

70. Pereira, A.C., Huddleston, D.E., Brickman, A.M., Sosunov, A.A., Hen, R., McKhann, G.M., Sloan, R., Gage, F.H., Brown, T.R., and Small, S.A. An in vivo correlate of exercise-induced neurogenesis in the adult dentate gyrus. *Proceedings of the National Academy of Science*, 104(13):5638–5643, 2007.

71. Christie B.R., Eadie, B.D., Kannangara, T.S., Robillard, J.M., Shin, J., and Titterness, A.K. Exercising our brains: How physical activity impacts synaptic plasticity in the dentate gyrus. *Neuromolecular Medicine*, 10(2):47–58, 2008.

72. Pereira, A.C., Huddleston, D.E., Brickman, A.M., Sosunov, A.A., Hen, R., McKhann, G.M., Sloan, R., Gage, F.H., Brown, T.R., and Small, S.A. An in vivo correlate of exercise-induced neurogenesis in the adult dentate gyrus. *Proceedings of the National Academy of Science*, 104(13):5638–5643, 2007.

73. Francis, K.T. The role of endorphins in exercise: A review of current knowledge. *Journal of Orthopaedic and Sports Physical Therapy*, 4(3):169–173, 1983.

74. Boecker, H., Sprenger, T., Spilker, M.E., Henriksen, G., Koppenhoefer, M., Wagner, K.J., Valet, M., Berthele, A., and Tolle, T.R. The runner's high: Opioidergic mechanisms in the human brain. *Cerebral Cortex*, 18(11):2523–2531, 2008.

75. Saanijoki, T., Tuominen, L., Tuulari, J.J., Nummenmaa, L., Arponen, E., Kalliokoski, K., and Hirvonen, J. Opioid release after high-intensity interval training in healthy human subjects. *Neuropsychopharmacology*, 43(2):246–254, 2018.

76. Raichlen, D.A., Foster, A.D., Gerdeman, G.L., Seillier, A., and Giuffrida, A. Wired to run: Exercise-induced endocannabinoid signaling in humans and cursorial mammals with implications for the "runner's high." *Journal of Experimental Biology*, 215:1331–1336, 2012.

77. Murray, R.F., Asghari, A., Egorov, D.D., Rutkowski, S.B., Siddall, P.J., Soden, R.J., and Ruff, R. Impact of spinal cord injury on self-perceived pre- and postmorbid cognitive, emotional and physical functioning. *Spinal Cord*, 45(6):429–436, 2007.

78. Craig, A., Guest, R., Tran, Y., and Middleton, J. Cognitive impairment and mood states after spinal cord injury. *Journal of Neurotrauma*, 34(6):1156–1163, 2017.

79. Chiaravalloti, N.D., Weber, E., Wylie, G., Dyson-Hudson, T., and Wecht, J.M. Patterns of cognitive deficits in persons with spinal cord injury as compared with both age-matched and older individuals without spinal cord injury. *Journal of Spinal Cord Medicine*, 43(1):88–97, 2020.

80. Sachdeva, R., Gao, F., Chan, C.C.H., and Krassioukov, A.V. Cognitive function after spinal cord injury: A systematic review. *Neurology*, 91:611–621, 2018.

81. Craig, A., Guest, R., Tran, Y., and Middleton, J. Cognitive impairment and mood states after spinal cord injury. *Journal of Neurotrauma*, 34(6):1156–1163, 2017.

82. Migliorini, C., Tonge, B., and Taleporos, G. Spinal cord injury and mental health. *Australian and New Zealand Journal of Psychiatry*, 42(4):309–314, 2008.

Chapter 3: Mind

1. Netz, Y., Wu, M.J., Becker, B.J., and Tenenbaum, G. Physical activity and psychological well-being in advanced age: A meta-analysis of intervention studies. *Psychology and Aging*, 20(2):272–284, 2005.

2. Greenleaf, C., Gould, D., and Dieffenbach, K. Factors influencing Olympic performance: Interviews with Atlanta and Nagano US Olympians. *Journal of Applied Sport Psychology*, 13(2):154–184, 2001.

3. Scully, D., Kremer, J., Meade, M.M., Graham, R., and Dudgeon, K. Physical exercise and psychological well being: A critical review. *British Journal of Sports Medicine*, 32(2):111–120, 1998.

4. Desharnais, R., Jobin, J., Côté, C., Lévesque, L., and Godin, G. Aerobic exercise and the placebo effect: A controlled study. *Psychosomatic Medicine*, 55(2):149–154, 1993.

5. Johnson, M. *The Meaning of the Body: Aesthetics of Human Understanding.* Chicago, IL: University of Chicago Press, 2007.

6. Prioreschi, P. *A History of Medicine: Volume II: Greek Medicine.* Omaha, NE: Horatius Press, 1996.

7. Cicero, M.T. *Cato Major: Or, A Treatise On Old Age.* Charleston, SC: Nabu Press, 2011.

8. Thoreau, H.D. *A Year in Thoreau's Journal: 1851.* New York: Penguin Classics, 1993.

9. Thelen, E., and Smith, L.B. *A Dynamic Systems Approach to the Development of Cognition and Action.* Cambridge, MA: MIT Press.

10. Miles, L.K., Nind, L.K., and Macrae, C.N. Moving through time. *Psychological Science*, 21(2):222–243, 2010.

11. Barsalou, L.W., Niedenthal, P.M., Barbey, A.K., and Ruppert, J.A. Social embodiment. In: Ross, B. (Ed.). *The Psychology of Learning and Motivation: Volume 43*. San Diego, CA: Academic Press, 43–92, 2003.

12. Niedenthal, P.M., Barsalou, L.W., Winkielman, P., Krauth-Gruber, S., and Ric, F. Embodiment in attitudes, social perception, and emotion. *Personality and Social Psychology Review*, 9(3):184–211, 2005.

13. Thomas, W., and Schubert, T.W. The power in your hand: Gender differences in bodily feedback from making a fist. *Personality and Social Psychology Bulletin*, 30(6):757–769, 2004.

14. Tiedens, L.Z., and Fragale, A.R. Power moves: Complementarity in dominant and submissive nonverbal behavior. *Journal of Personality and Social Psychology*, 84(3):558–568, 2003.

15. Jostmann, N.B., Lakens, D., and Schubert, T.W. Weight as an embodiment of importance. *Psychological Science*, 20(9):1169–1174, 2009.

16. Bhalla, M., and Proffitt, D.R. Visual-motor recalibration in geographical slant perception. *Journal of Experimental Psychology: Human Perception and Performance*, 25(4):1076–1096, 1999.

17. Proffitt, D.R., Stefanucci, J., Banton, T., and Epstein, W. The role of effort in perceiving distance. *Physiological Science*, 14(2):106–112, 2003.

18. Proffitt, D.R. Embodied perception and the economy of action. *Perspectives on Psychological Science*, 1(2):110–122, 2006.

19. Proffitt, D.R., Stefanucci, J., Banton, T., and Epstein, W. The role of effort in perceiving distance. *Physiological Science*, 14(2):106–112, 2003.

20. Hayes, D., and Ross, C.E. Body and mind: The effect of exercise, overweight, and physical health on psychological well-being. *Journal of Health and Social Behavior*, 27(4):387–400, 1986.

21. Sheline, Y.I., Wang, P.W., Gado, M.H., Csernansky, J.G., and Vannier, M.W. Hippocampal atrophy in recurrent major depression. *Proceedings of the National Academy of Sciences*, 93:3908–3913, 1996.

22. Banasr, M., Dwyer, J.M., and Duman, R.S. Cell atrophy and loss in depression: Reversal by antidepressant treatment. *Current Opinion in Cell Biology*, 23(6):730–737, 2011.

23. Santarelli, L., Saxe, M., Gross, C., Surget, A., Battaglia, F., Dulawa, S., Weisstaub, N., Lee, J., Duman, R., Arancio, O., Belzung, C., and Hen, R. Requirement of hippocampal neurogenesis for the behavioral effects of antidepressants. *Science*, 301(5634):805–809, 2003.

24. Santarelli, L., Saxe, M., Gross, C., Surget, A., Battaglia, F., Dulawa, S., Weisstaub, N., Lee, J., Duman, R., Arancio, O., Belzung, C., and Hen, R. Requirement of hippocampal neurogenesis for the behavioral effects of antidepressants. *Science*, 301(5634):805–809, 2003.

25. Carek, P.J., Laibstain, S.E., and Carek, S.M. Exercise for the treatment of depression and anxiety. *International Journal of Psychiatry in Medicine*, 41(1):15–28, 2011.

26. Ernst, C., Olson, A.K., Pinel, J.P.J., Lam, R.W., and Christie, B.R. Anti-depressant effects of exercise: Evidence for an adult-neurogenesis hypothesis? *Journal of Psychiatry & Neuroscience*, 31(2):84–92, 2006.

27. Taylor, M.K., Markham, A.E., Reis, J.P., Padilla, G.A., Potterat, E.G., Drummond, S.P.A., and Mujica-Parodi, L.R. Physical fitness influences stress reactions to extreme military training. *Military Medicine*, 173(8):738–742, 2008.

28. Ruo, B., Rumsfeld, J.S., Pipkin, S., and Whooley, M.A. Relation between depressive symptoms and treadmill exercise capacity in the Heart and Soul Study. *American Journal of Cardiology*, 94(1):96–99, 2004.

29. Yau, S.Y., Li, A., Hoo, R.L.C., Ching, Y.P., Christie, B.R., Lee, T.M.C., Xu, A., and So, K-F. Physical exercise-induced hippocampal neurogenesis and antidepressant effects are mediated by the adipocyte hormone adiponectin. *Proceedings of the National Academy of Sciences*, 111(44):15810–15815, 2014.

30. Childs, E., and de Wit, H. Regular exercise is associated with emotional resilience to acute stress in healthy adults. *Frontiers in Physiology*, 5:161, 2014.

31. Klaperski, S., von Dawans, B., Heinrichs, M., and Fuchs, R. Does the level of physical exercise affect physiological and psychological responses to psycho-social stress in women? *Psychology of Sport and Exercise*, 14:266–274, 2013.

32. Zschucke, E., Renneberg, B., Dimeo, F., Wüstenberg, T., and Ströhle, A. The stress-buffering effect of acute exercise: Evidence for HPA axis negative feedback. *Psychoneuroendocrinology*, 51:414–425, 2015.

33. Klaperski, S., von Dawans, B., Heinrichs, M., and Fuchs, R. Effects of a 12-week endurance training program on the physiological response to psy-chosocial stress in men: A randomized controlled trial. *Journal of Behavioral Medicine*, 37(6):1118–1133, 2014.

34. Deuster, P.A., and Silverman, M.N. Physical fitness: A pathway to health and resilience. *US Army Medical Department Journal*, Oct.–Dec.:24–35, 2013.

35. Roth, D.L., and Holmes, D.S. Influence of physical fitness in determining the impact of stressful life events on physical and psychologic health. *Psychosomatic Medicine*, 47(2):164–173, 1985.

36. Silverman, M.N., and Deuster, P.A. Biological mechanisms underlying the role of physical fitness in health and resilience. *Interface Focus*, 4(5):20140040, 2014.

37. Greenwood, B.N., and Fleshner, M. Exercise, learned helplessness, and the stress-resistant brain. *Neuromolecular Medicine*, 10:81–98, 2008.

38. Tillage, R.P., Wilson, G.E., Liles, L.C., Holmes, P.V., and Weinshenker, D. Chronic environmental or genetic elevation of galanin in noradrenergic neu-rons confers stress resilience in mice. *Journal of Neuroscience*, 40(39):7464–7474, 2020.

39. Martikainen, S., Pesonen, A.K., Lahti, J., Heinonen, K., Feldt, K., Pyhälä, R., Tammelin, T., Kajantie, E., Eriksson, J.G., Strandberg, T.E., and Räikkönen, K. Higher levels of physical activity are associated with lower hypothalamic-pituitary-adrenocortical axis reactivity to psychosocial stress in children. *Journal of Clinical Endocrinology and Metabolism*, 98(4):E619–E627, 2013.

40. Perchtold-Stefan, C.M., Fink, A., Rominger, C., Weiss, E.M., and Papousek, I. More habitual physical activity is linked to the use of specific, more adaptive cognitive reappraisal strategies in dealing with stressful events. *Stress and Health*, 36(3):274–286, 2020.

41. Papousek, I., Weiss, E.M., Perchtold, C.M., Weber, H., Assuncao, V.L., Schulter, G., Lackner, H.K., and Fink, A. The capacity for generating cognitive reappraisals is reflected in asymmetric activation of frontal brain regions. *Brain Imaging and Behavior*, 11:577–590, 2017.

42. Watkins, T., and Umphress, E.E. Strong body, clear mind: Physical activity diminishes the effects of supervisor interpersonal injustice. *Personnel Psychology*, 73:641–667, 2020.

43. Aitchison, C., Turner, L.A., Ansley, L., Thompson, K.G., Micklewright, D., and St. Clair Gibson, A. Inner dialogue and its relationship to perceived exertion during different running intensities. *Perceptual and Motor Skills*, 117(1):1053–1072, 2013.

44. Tammen, V.V. Elite middle and long distance runners associative/dissociative coping. *Journal of Applied Sport Psychology*, 8:1–8, 1996.

45. Scheef, L., Jankowski, J., Daamen, M., Weyer, G., Klingenberg, M., Renner, J., Mueckter, S., Schürmann, B., Musshoff, F., Wagner, M., Schild, H.H., Zimmer, A., and Boecker, H. An fMRI study on the acute effects of exercise on pain processing in trained athletes. *Pain*, 153(8):1702–1714, 2012.

Chapter 4: Endurance

1. Bramble, D.M., and Lieberman, D.E. Endurance running and the evolution of *Homo*. *Nature*, 432(7015):345–352, 2004.

2. Ekblom, B., and Hermansen, L. Cardiac output in athletes. *Journal of Applied Physiology*, 25(5):619–625, 1968.

3. Niedermeier, M., Einwanger, J., Hartl, A., and Kopp, M. Affective responses in mountain hiking—A randomized crossover trial focusing on differences between indoor and outdoor activity. *PLOS ONE*, 12(5):e0177719, 2017.

4. Bratman, G.N., Hamilton, J.P., Hahn, K.S., Daily, G.C., and Gross, J.J. Nature experience reduces rumination and subgenual prefrontal cortex activation. *Proceedings of the National Academy of Sciences*, 112(28):8567–8572, 2015.

Chapter 5: Strength

1. Herzog, W. Muscle. In: Nigg, B.M., and Herzog, W. (Eds.). *Biomechanics of the Musculo-skeletal System*. Toronto: Wiley, 2007, 169–217.

2. Boccia, G., Pizzigalli, L., Formicola, D., Ivaldi, M., and Rainoldi, A. Higher neuromuscular manifestations of fatigue in dynamic than isometric pull-up tasks in rock climbers. *Journal of Human Kinetics*, 47:31–39, 2015.

Chapter 7: Cognitive Flexibility
1. Scharfen, H.-E., and Memmert, D. The relationship between cognitive functions and sport-specific motor skills in elite youth soccer players. *Frontiers in Psychology*, 10:817, 2019.

Index

About the Author

It started with a race around the track in sixth grade in Marlboro, New Jersey. Little did Jason know how much it would define his career and life. A Brooklyn, New York, native (you can take the boy out of Brooklyn but you can't take Brooklyn out of the boy), he grew up playing baseball and soccer and running track. It was intoxicating. The passion that Jason found as a kid for the science of athletic performance (one of his earliest questions was how baseball pitchers throw curve balls) placed him on a yellow brick road that he still follows as a coach, exercise physiologist, author, speaker, and creator of the REVO$_2$LUTION RUNNING™ certification program for coaches and fitness professionals. He is also founder and CEO of the women's specialty run-coaching company Kyniska Running, LLC.

A TEDx speaker, Dr. Karp has given hundreds of international lectures and has been a featured speaker at most of the world's top fitness conferences and coaching clinics, including Asia Fitness Convention, Indonesia Fitness & Health Expo, FILEX Fitness Convention (Australia), US Track & Field and Cross Country Coaches Association Convention, American College of Sports Medicine Conference, IDEA World Fitness Convention, SCW Fitness MANIA, National Strength & Conditioning Association Conference, and CanFitPro, among others. He has been an instructor for USA Track & Field's level 3 coaching certification and for coaching camps at the US Olympic Training Center.

At age 24, Dr. Karp became one of the youngest college head coaches in the country, leading the Georgian Court University women's cross-country team in New Jersey to the regional championship and winning honors as NAIA Northeast Region Coach of the Year. As a high school track and field and cross-country coach, he has produced state qualifiers and All-Americans. He currently coaches a wide variety of runners.

A prolific writer, Dr. Karp is the author of eleven other books: *Running Periodization, The Inner Runner, Running a Marathon For Dummies, Lose It Forever, Run Your Fat Off, Sexercise, 14-Minute Metabolic Workouts, Running for Women, 101 Winning Racing Strategies for Runners, 101 Developmental Concepts & Workouts for Cross Country Runners,* and *How to Survive Your PhD.* He is also editor of the sixth edition of *Track & Field Omnibook.* He has more than 400 articles published in numerous international coaching, running, and fitness trade and consumer magazines, including *Track Coach, Techniques for Track & Field and Cross Country, New Studies in Athletics, Runner's World, Running Times, Women's Running, Marathon & Beyond, IDEA Fitness Journal, Oxygen, PTontheNet.com,* and *Shape,* among others. He also served as senior editor for Active Network.

Dr. Karp is a USA Track & Field certified coach, has been sponsored by PowerBar and Brooks, and was a member of the silver-medal winning US Masters team at the 2013 World Maccabiah Games in Israel.

For his work and contributions to his industry, he was awarded the 2011 IDEA Personal Trainer of the Year (the fitness industry's highest award), is a two-time recipient of the President's Council on Sports, Fitness & Nutrition Community Leadership Award (2014, 2019), and was a 2019 finalist for Personal Fitness Professional Trainer of the Year and 2020 finalist for Association of Fitness Studios Influencer of the Year.